# OTHER FAST FACTS BOOKS

Fast Facts on **ADOLESCENT HEALTH FOR NURSING AND HEALTH PROFESSIONALS**: A Care Guide *(Herrman)*

Fast Facts for the **ANTEPARTUM AND POSTPARTUM NURSE**: A Nursing Orientation and Care Guide *(Davidson)*

Fast Facts Workbook for **CARDIAC DYSRHYTHMIAS AND 12-LEAD EKGs** *(Desmarais)*

Fast Facts for the **CARDIAC SURGERY NURSE**: Caring for Cardiac Surgery Patients, Third Edition *(Hodge)*

Fast Facts for **CAREER SUCCESS IN NURSING**: Making the Most of Mentoring *(Vance)*

Fast Facts for the **CATH LAB NURSE** *(McCulloch)*

Fast Facts for the **CLASSROOM NURSING INSTRUCTOR**: Classroom Teaching *(Yoder-Wise, Kowalski)*

Fast Facts for the **CLINICAL NURSE LEADER** *(Wilcox, Deerhake)*

Fast Facts for the **CLINICAL NURSE MANAGER**: Managing a Changing Workplace, Second Edition *(Fry)*

Fast Facts for the **CLINICAL NURSING INSTRUCTOR**: Clinical Teaching, Third Edition *(Kan, Stabler-Haas)*

Fast Facts on **COMBATING NURSE BULLYING, INCIVILITY, AND WORKPLACE VIOLENCE**: What Nurses Need to Know *(Ciocco)*

Fast Facts for the **CRITICAL CARE NURSE**, Second Edition *(Hewett)*

Fast Facts About **CURRICULUM DEVELOPMENT IN NURSING**: How to Develop and Evaluate Educational Programs, Second Edition *(McCoy, Anema)*

Fast Facts for **DEMENTIA CARE**: What Nurses Need to Know, Second Edition *(Miller)*

Fast Facts for **DEVELOPING A NURSING ACADEMIC PORTFOLIO**: What You Really Need to Know *(Wittmann-Price)*

Fast Facts for **DNP ROLE DEVELOPMENT**: A Career Navigation Guide *(Menonna-Quinn, Tortorella Genova)*

Fast Facts About **EKGs FOR NURSES**: The Rules of Identifying EKGs *(Landrum)*

Fast Facts for the **ER NURSE**: Emergency Department Orientation, Third Edition *(Buettner)*

Fast Facts for **EVIDENCE-BASED PRACTICE IN NURSING**: Third Edition *(Godshall)*

Fast Facts for the **FAITH COMMUNITY NURSE**: Implementing FCN/Parish Nursing *(Hickman)*

Fast Facts About **FORENSIC NURSING**: What You Need to Know *(Scannell)*

Fast Facts for the **GERONTOLOGY NURSE**: A Nursing Care Guide *(Eliopoulos)*

Fast Facts About **GI AND LIVER DISEASES FOR NURSES**: What APRNs Need to Know *(Chaney)*

Fast Facts About the **GYNECOLOGICAL EXAM**: A Professional Guide for NPs, PAs, and Midwives, Second Edition *(Secor, Fantasia)*

Fast Facts in **HEALTH INFORMATICS FOR NURSES** *(Hardy)*

Fast Facts for **HEALTH PROMOTION IN NURSING**: Promoting Wellness *(Miller)*

Fast Facts for Nurses About **HOME INFUSION THERAPY**: The Expert's Best Practice Guide *(Gorski)*

Fast Facts for the **HOSPICE NURSE**: A Concise Guide to End-of-Life Care, Second Edition *(Wright)*

Fast Facts for the **L&D NURSE**: Labor & Delivery Orientation, Second Edition *(Groll)*

Fast Facts for the **LONG-TERM CARE NURSE**: What Nursing Home and Assisted Living Nurses Need to Know *(Eliopoulos)*

Fast Facts to **LOVING YOUR RESEARCH PROJECT**: A Stress-Free Guide for Novice Researchers in Nursing and Healthcare *(Marshall)*

Fast Facts for **MAKING THE MOST OF YOUR CAREER IN NURSING** *(Redulla)*

Fast Facts for **MANAGING PATIENTS WITH A PSYCHIATRIC DISORDER**: What RNs, NPs, and New Psych Nurses Need to Know *(Marshall)*

Fast Facts About **MEDICAL CANNABIS AND OPIOIDS**: Minimizing Opioid Use Through Cannabis *(Smith, Smith)*

Fast Facts for the **MEDICAL OFFICE NURSE**: What You Really Need to Know *(Richmeier)*

Fast Facts for the **MEDICAL–SURGICAL NURSE**: Clinical Orientation *(Ciocco)*

Fast Facts for the **NEONATAL NURSE**: A Nursing Orientation and Care Guide *(Davidson)*

Fast Facts About **NEUROCRITICAL CARE**: A Quick Reference for the Advanced Practice Provider *(McLaughlin)*

Fast Facts for the **NEW NURSE PRACTITIONER**: What You Really Need to Know, Second Edition *(Aktan)*

Fast Facts for **NURSE PRACTITIONERS:** Practice Essentials for Clinical Subspecialties *(Aktan)*

Fast Facts for the **NURSE PRECEPTOR**: Keys to Providing a Successful Preceptorship *(Ciocco)*

Fast Facts for the **NURSE PSYCHOTHERAPIST**: The Process of Becoming *(Jones, Tusaie)*

Fast Facts About **NURSING AND THE LAW**: Law for Nurses *(Grant, Ballard)*

Fast Facts About the **NURSING PROFESSION**: Historical Perspectives *(Hunt)*

Fast Facts for the **OPERATING ROOM NURSE**: An Orientation and Care Guide, Second Edition *(Criscitelli)*

Fast Facts for the **PEDIATRIC NURSE**: An Orientation Guide *(Rupert, Young)*

Fast Facts Handbook for **PEDIATRIC PRIMARY CARE:** A Guide for Nurse Practitioners and Physician Assistants *(Ruggiero, Ruggiero)*

Fast Facts About **PRESSURE ULCER CARE FOR NURSES**: How to Prevent, Detect, and Resolve Them *(Dziedzic)*

Fast Facts About **PTSD**: A Guide for Nurses and Other Health Care Professionals *(Adams)*

Fast Facts for the **RADIOLOGY NURSE**: An Orientation and Nursing Care Guide, Second Edition *(Grossman)*

Fast Facts About **RELIGION FOR NURSES**: Implications for Patient Care *(Taylor)*

Fast Facts for the **SCHOOL NURSE**: What You Need to Know, Third Edition *(Loschiavo)*

Fast Facts About **SEXUALLY TRANSMITTED INFECTIONS**: A Nurse's Guide to Expert Patient Care *(Scannell)*

Fast Facts for **STROKE CARE NURSING**: An Expert Care Guide, Second Edition *(Morrison)*

Fast Facts for the **STUDENT NURSE**: Nursing Student Success *(Stabler-Haas)*

Fast Facts About **SUBSTANCE USE DISORDERS**: What Every Nurse, APRN, and PA Needs to Know *(Marshall, Spencer)*

Fast Facts for the **TRAVEL NURSE**: Travel Nursing *(Landrum)*

Fast Facts for the **TRIAGE NURSE**: An Orientation and Care Guide, Second Edition *(Visser, Montejano)*

Fast Facts for the **WOUND CARE NURSE**: Practical Wound Management *(Kifer)*

Fast Facts for **WRITING THE DNP PROJECT**: Effective Structure, Content, and Presentation *(Christenbery)*

# Forthcoming FAST FACTS Books

Fast Facts for the **ADULT-GERONTOLOGY ACUTE CARE NURSE PRACTITIONER** *(Carpenter)*

Fast Facts About **COMPETENCY-BASED EDUCATION IN NURSING**: How to Teach Competency Mastery *(Wittmann-Price, Gittings)*

Fast Facts for **CREATING A SUCCESSFUL TELEHEALTH SERVICE**: A How-to Guide for Nurse Practitioners *(Heidesch)*

Fast Facts About **DIVERSITY, EQUITY, AND INCLUSION** *(Davis)*

Fast Facts for the **ER NURSE**: Guide to a Successful Emergency Department Orientation, Fourth Edition *(Buettner)*

Fast Facts for the **L&D NURSE**: Labor & Delivery Orientation, Third Edition *(Groll)*

Fast Facts About **LGBTQ CARE FOR NURSES** *(Traister)*

Fast Facts for the **NEONATAL NURSE**: Care Essentials for Normal and High-Risk Neonates, Second Edition *(Davidson)*

Fast Facts for the **NURSE PRECEPTOR**: Keys to Providing a Successful Preceptorship, Second Edition *(Ciocco)*

Fast Facts for **PATIENT SAFETY IN NURSING** *(Hunt)*

**Visit www.springerpub.com to order.**

*FAST FACTS* for
# THE NURSE PRECEPTOR

**Maggie Ciocco, MS, RN, BC** is currently a nursing program advisor. She has over 30 years of experience in nursing education, including as a preceptor, mentor, staff development instructor, orientation coordinator, nursing lab instructor, clinical instructor, and program advisor. Ms. Ciocco received her MS in nursing from Syracuse University, her BS in nursing from Seton Hall University, and her AAS from Ocean County College in Toms River, New Jersey. She has been an American Nurses Credentialing Center board-certified medical–surgical nurse for nearly 30 years. Throughout her years as an educator, she has established preceptorship programs in acute, subacute, and long-term care settings. She is a member of the National League for Nursing. Ms. Ciocco was awarded the Sigma Theta Tau–Lambda Delta chapter Hannelore Sweetwood Mentor of the Year award in 2012. She is the author of *Fast Facts for the Medical–Surgical Nurse: Clinical Orientation in a Nutshell*, published by Springer Publishing Company in 2014 as well as *Fast Facts on Combating Nurse Bullying, Incivility and Workplace Violence*, published by Springer Publishing Company in 2018.

*FAST FACTS* for
# THE NURSE PRECEPTOR

## Keys to Providing a Successful Preceptorship

**Second Edition**

Maggie Ciocco, MS, RN, BC

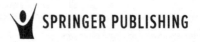

SPRINGER PUBLISHING

Springer Publishing Company, LLC
11 West 42nd Street, New York, NY 10036
www.springerpub.com
connect.springerpub.com/

*Acquisitions Editor*: Rachel X. Landes
*Compositor*: Amnet Systems

*ISBN*: 978-0-8261-3601-5
*ebook ISBN*: 978-0-8261-3612-1
*DOI*: 10.1891/9780826136121

20 21 22 23/ 5 4 3 2 1

**Library of Congress Cataloging-in-Publication Data**
Names: Ciocco, Margaret Curry, author.
Title: Fast facts for the nurse preceptor : keys to providing a successful
  preceptorship / Maggie Ciocco.
Other titles: Fast facts (Springer Publishing Company)
Description: Second edition. | New York, NY : Springer Publishing Company,
  LLC, [2021] | Series: Fast facts | Includes bibliographical references
  and index. |
Identifiers: LCCN 2020027537 (print) | LCCN 2020027538 (ebook) | ISBN
  9780826136015 (paperback) | ISBN 9780826136121 (ebook)
Subjects: MESH: Education, Nursing | Preceptorship—methods |
  Preceptorship—standards | Students, Nursing—psychology | Staff
  Development—methods | Clinical Competence
Classification: LCC RT74.7 (print) | LCC RT74.7 (ebook) | NLM WY 18 |
  DDC 610.73071/1—dc23
LC record available at https://lccn.loc.gov/2020027537
LC ebook record available at https://lccn.loc.gov/2020027538

*This book is dedicated to my family . . .*
*thank you for your patience and love.*
*To Benjamin James, Ophelia Grace, and P. Nicholas,*
*love you to the stars and back!*

*This book is also dedicated to all preceptors . . .*
*remember, you model the future of nursing.*

# Contents

*Foreword*   Linda J. Hassler, MS, RN, GCNS-BC, FNGNA                    *xi*
*Preface*                                                                *xiii*

## Part I  INTRODUCTION TO THE ROLE OF THE PRECEPTOR

1.  Preceptorship in a Nutshell                                          3

2.  Selection, Education, and Retention of the Preceptor                 15

3.  Preceptee Learning and Preceptor Teaching Styles                     27

4.  The Challenging Student                                              39

5.  Critical Thinking Skills                                            49

6.  Organizing the Clinical Day                                          63

## Part II  COMPONENTS OF EFFECTIVE PRECEPTORSHIP

7.  Prioritization and Communication                                     77

8.  The Value of Feedback                                               91

9.  The Art of Delegation                                               105

10. Precepting the Accelerated BSN and Advanced
    Practice Registered Nurse (APRN)                                     115

11. Recognizing and Helping the Preceptee
Who Is Struggling                                             127

12. The Unsafe Preceptee and How to Avoid "Failure to Fail"    139

### Part III PREPARING THE PRECEPTEE FOR THE FUTURE

13. Conflict Resolution and Bullying in Nursing               153

14. Helping the Preceptee Deal With Reality Shock             163

15. Preparing for the Future                                  173

### Part IV PROBLEM-SOLVING AND CLINICAL TOOLS

16. Preceptorship Competency Forms and Clinical Tools         189

17. Concerns of the Preceptor and Case Studies               201

Index                                                        213

# Foreword

Maggie Ciocco's *Fast Facts for the Nurse Preceptor, Second Edition: Keys to Providing a Successful Preceptorship* is one book you will want to crack open today! It is full of practical how-to guidance, evidence-based resources, and references for further reading, and it is a must-read for any nurse who has been a preceptor or may become a preceptor.

Ms. Ciocco unlocks what every new nurse preceptor needs to know to be successful with a preceptee, whether the preceptee is a nursing student in their final semester or a new nurse on orientation. The book covers everything necessary in a fast, factual, easy-to-read format. However, you do not have to be a new preceptor to benefit from it.

Many of us have had the misfortune of being "tagged" to be a preceptor without any formal nurse preceptor education. This book is a great resource for these seasoned nurses as well, with its comprehensive review of basics like shift organization, prioritization, communication, delegation, and conflict resolution. It also covers the dreaded reality shock that new nurses will face after the honeymoon phase, how to recognize those who are struggling, how to encourage critical thinking, and how to prepare for the future when the preceptorship is over. Throughout the book, Ms. Ciocco gives great examples of problem-solving dos and don'ts, checklists, and forms.

*Fast Facts for the Nurse Preceptor* is also an excellent resource for educators looking to implement nurse preceptor programs in their workplaces, and a great textbook for preceptor students.

**Linda J. Hassler, MS, RN, GCNS-BC, FNGNA**
*Project Director*
*New Jersey Action Coalition Nurse*
*Residency in Long Term Care Program*

# Preface

As a nurse preceptor, it is your professional obligation to ensure that a preceptorship of the highest standard is provided. A high-quality preceptorship will help to ensure that the nurse or student, hereafter known as the preceptee, will deliver quality, patient-centered care that is safe and has its foundation in evidence-based practice.

Many healthcare agencies and research bodies have conducted studies regarding the healthcare system in the United States. Two major themes have emerged from their work: issues of quality and safety, and their pertinence to professional nursing practice.

In its year 2000 report *To Err is Human: Building a Safer Health System,* The National Academies of Science, Engineering and Medicine (The National Academies), formerly known as the Institute of Medicine or IOM, revealed as many as 98,000 Americans die every year as a result of errors in their care. As horrifying as that number is, the exact number is indeterminable due to study methods and could actually be in the hundreds of thousands with an equally high number of unnecessary patient injuries.

For generations, healthcare workers from all disciplines have been taught in their independent "silos," meaning they learn only what their discipline entails without learning about the other disciplines and their roles in the care of the patient (Hendricson & Kleffner, 2002). The *To Err is Human* report explicitly stated this could be leading to patient care errors and deaths. Healthcare education, the report states, relies on this "silo" education, with students being passive in their education. They are unable to integrate knowledge with assessment of the patient condition; they are unable to be adequately vigilant against errors in care; and they are unable to make patient care decisions when faced with a problem. Entry-level professionals lack training in the electronic medical record or with information management systems, so they rely on memorization of facts rather than current, up-to-date knowledge. During their basic education and preceptorship, these new professionals also lacked opportunities to practice problem-solving skills.

That report was followed in 2001 with *Crossing the Quality Chasm: A New Health System for the 21st Century*, which "identified health care quality issues, called for a radical redesign of the U.S. health care system and proposed six quality outcomes: safety, effectiveness, patient centeredness, timeliness, efficiency and quality" (Ulrich, 2011). In 2003, The National Academies published *Health Professions Education: A Bridge to Quality*, which introduced a core set of competencies to integrate into the education of all healthcare professions. In 2004, in response to a request from the Agency for Healthcare Research and Quality (AHRQ), The National Academies published a report that addressed the role of nursing and the healthcare environment and their effects on patient safety. In 2007, the Robert Wood Johnson Foundation (RWJF) supported a program called Quality and Safety Education for Nurses (QSEN) to address "the challenge of preparing nurses with the competencies necessary to continuously improve the quality of safety of the health care systems in which they work" (Ulrich, 2011). The QSEN team adopted competencies developed by The National Academies and outlined the knowledge and skills for each competency. They are now utilized throughout areas in which nurses are educated and practice. They include:

- That nurses should recognize the patient as a full partner in their care (patient-centered care)
- That nurses should be offered the opportunity to be full members of the healthcare team, able to openly communicate and share in the decision-making to ensure quality patient care (teamwork and collaboration)
- That all care provided should be based on the most current standards (evidence-based practice)
- That patient care data should be collected and monitored to ensure that the outcomes of care and patient safety standards are continually improved (quality improvement)

- That the risk of harm to a patient is minimized (safety)
- That information and technology is used to communicate among healthcare professionals in order to lessen the chance for error, collect data, support decision-making (informatics), and allow for continuing facility-based education

In 2008, the RWJF collaborated with The National Academies and instituted the two-year RWJF Initiative on the Future of Nursing. The goal of the collaboration was to study the possibility of encouraging the profession of nursing to meet the needs of the public in the changing atmosphere of healthcare. The report produced by the committee, *The Future of Nursing: Leading Change, Advancing Health*, made recommendations for nurse training, education, professional leadership, and workforce policy. Many of the recommendations continue to have a direct impact on nursing education and preceptorship:

- Implement nurse residency programs
- Increase the proportion of nurses with a baccalaureate degree to 80% by 2020. (As of 2019 it is predicted that this goal will not be met as only 56% of nurses possessed a BSN in 2017.)
- Double the number of nurses with doctoral degrees by 2020. (As of 2019, this goal was noted to be achieved with 28,000 doctoral prepared nurses in the United States.)
- Ensure that nurses engage in lifelong learning
- Prepare and enable nurses to lead change to advance health

The full list of recommendations and how they are being implemented on a state and national basis can be found at http://thefutureofnursing.org.

So how have we done? Nearly 20 years after the publication of *To Err is Human: Building a Safer Healthcare System*, the improvement in patient safety has been slow and limited. Patients continue to face harm when admitted to a hospital or other healthcare facility. Barriers to patient safety continue to exist. It doesn't matter how many studies and reports are published if short staffing, poor documentation, poor handover reporting, and a lack of critical thinking continue to exist. Patients will continue to suffer injury and death.

Major patient safety issues continue to occur throughout the healthcare system. These include:

- Medication errors—Despite new technology that includes barcoding of medication and computerized verification of allergies, dosage range, and order entry, medication errors, previously thought to be decreasing, may actually be increasing due to staff workarounds and lack of education regarding the benefits of safety measures.

- Surgical injuries—Multiple safety measures have been implemented, but their success in decreasing injuries is contingent upon correct utilization by medical and nursing staff, which does not always occur.

- Other errors including poor communication among staff at change-of-shift report, unit handoff, failure to rescue, patient falls, decubitus ulcers, and improper identification of staff, many with dire consequences.

Even though hospitals were successful in implementing measures to decrease infection rates for patients with central lines, ventilators, and urinary catheters, infection rates continue to remain high. This is thought to be due to staff inconsistently utilizing infection prevention techniques such as proper handwashing. Healthcare facilities continually struggle with implementing new safety measures while older safety measures that are not successful remain in place. Patient safety is a direct result of a culture-wide acceptance and implementation of education and standards.

The goal of this text is to present a foundation for preceptorship of newly graduated registered professional nurses from traditional and accelerated programs, student nurses. Students from NP programs are briefly reviewed as well.

*Quality* and *safety* are paramount issues in nursing practice. It is because of this that they should be emphasized throughout nursing education and preceptorship.

**Maggie Ciocco**

## References

Institute of Medicine. (2001). *Crossing the quality chasm: A new health care system for the 21st century.* Washington, DC: The National Academies Press.

Institute of Medicine. (2003). *Health professions education: A bridge to quality.* Washington, DC: The National Academies Press.

Institute of Medicine & the Robert Wood Johnson Foundation. (2011). *Initiative on the future of nursing.* Retrieved from https://www .nursingworld.org/practice-policy/iom-future-of-nursing-report/

Hendricson, W. D., & Kleffner, J. H. (2002). Assessing and helping challenging students: Part One, why do some students have difficulty learning? *Journal of Dental Education, 66*(1), 43–61.

Ulrich, B. T. (2011). The preceptor role. In B. T. Ulrich (Ed.), *Mastering precepting: A nurse's handbook for success* (pp. 1–16). Indianapolis, IN: Sigma Theta Tau.

## Bibliography

Bates, D. W., & Singh, H. (2018). Two decades since to err is human: An assessment of progress and emerging priorities in patient safety. *Health Affairs, 37*(11). doi:10.1377/hlthaff.2018.0738

Federico, F. (2015, December 6). *15 years after to err is human: The status of patient safety in the US and UK*. Institute for Healthcare Improvement. Retrieved from http://www.ihi.org/communities/blogs/15-years-after-to-err-is-human-the-status-of-patient-safety-in-the-us-and-the-uk

Thew, J. (2017, October). *Goal of Nursing Workforce with 80% BSNS Unlikely by 2020*. Retrieved from https://www.healthleadersmedia.com/nursing/goal-nursing-workforce-80-bsns-unlikely-2020

# I

# Introduction to the Role of the Preceptor

# 1

# Preceptorship in a Nutshell

*A preceptor is many things: a teacher, a coach, a role model, a counselor. Being a preceptor to a student, graduate, or new nurse is one of the most important roles of an experienced nurse. Nursing students "consistently report that the biggest influence in developing critical thinking and establishing a strong nursing identity lies with their preceptor" (Maguire, Zambroski, & Cadena, 2012). Preceptorship is a very important time for both the new nurse and student, and for the nursing school, unit, or facility as well, because it lays the groundwork for future employees and their relationships within the facility as well as the continuing education of the nurse. Those who become preceptors should continually strive to educate themselves and hone their skills in order to be effective.*

After reading this chapter, the reader will be able to:

1. List five qualities of an ineffectual preceptor
2. List five qualities of an ideal preceptor
3. List 10 responsibilities of a mentor
4. List the phases of preceptorship
5. Describe the benefits of preceptorship

## THE INEFFECTUAL PRECEPTOR

The preceptorship of a nurse or student has far-reaching effects, influencing everything from the safety of the patient and the quality of care the patient receives to the employment, retention, and job satisfaction of the new nurse. If, when reading the following behaviors attributable to an ineffectual nursing preceptor, you notice that they reflect your teaching style, then take advantage of preceptor education. Recognize these behaviors can be changed but the most successful preceptors do not exhibit these qualities. You are an ineffectual preceptor if:

- You are unclear about the goals of orientation.
- You do not ascertain the preceptee's skill and knowledge level prior to the start of orientation.
- You do not ascertain the learning style of the preceptee and teach to it.
- You do not question the preceptee to determine if there are any patient care areas in which they feel weak (e.g., skills not experienced during nursing school or in a previous work experience).
- You do not introduce the preceptee to fellow team members and do not help the preceptee feel like part of the team.
- You do not orient the preceptee to the unit so that they know where items are located or typical procedures to follow.
- The goals and expectations for orientation are unclear and are not stated in writing.
- The goals you establish are not measurable or achievable.
- You do not review the goals for the day or for orientation with the preceptee.
- You are inconsistent in your communication style.
- You do not allow the preceptee time to practice skills prior to attempting them.
- You do not build new skills upon the current skill level.
- You delegate to the preceptee beyond their skill level or beyond their scope of practice.
- You do not seek out new learning experiences for the preceptee but instead allow the preceptee to find learning situations on their own.
- You fail to provide guidance in the completion of a new skill, assessment, or other nursing function.

- Your clinical skills and techniques are not evidence based or correct; you take shortcuts to save time, but, in doing so, may unknowingly endanger the patient. You pressure the preceptee to perform these skills as you do.
- You leave the preceptee alone during new patient care situations, endangering the patient.
- You allow the preceptee to do the work other staff does not wish to complete.
- You are continually rude to the preceptee, fellow staff, families, and patients.
- You allow the preceptee to experience a lot of "downtime," for example by allowing them to "hang around" the nurses' station rather than engaging in patient care or learning new skills.
- You frequently cancel scheduled meeting times with the preceptee, the unit manager, the unit educator, or faculty members, therefore allowing communication to break down among all parties.
- You allow the preceptee to be utilized as staff prior to the end of preceptorship.
- Act as a "friend" rather than a role model and teacher

### Fast Facts

The preceptorship experience will be remembered by the preceptee long after they have left the facility. How the preceptor conducts themselves and the orientation period will influence not only how the preceptee feels about the profession of nursing for years to come but also the quality of care their patients receive.

## YOU MIGHT BE A GREAT PRECEPTOR IF...

Preceptors affect how the preceptee "fits" (or does not fit) into unit society, as well as the preceptee's skill development (or lack thereof) and their proficient (or poor) patient care. A facility or nurse manager should never assume a registered nurse with excellent clinical skills will automatically translate those skills to this new arena by naturally performing as an effective preceptor. The preceptor has many roles and must be able to understand and conduct them all well.

The ideal preceptor is a teacher who:

- Provides learning and practice objectives that are concrete and measurable and in writing
- Assists the preceptee with establishing learning goals that are measurable and can be met within the confines of the precepting experience and assists in updating those goals as needed (hourly, daily, weekly, etc)
- Objectively assesses the learning needs of the preceptee
- Assists in the development of learning plans
- Understands the learning level of the student (first-year student, graduate nurse, experienced nurse but new to a unit, student nurse practitioner, etc.).
- Implements shared learning plans (facility and preceptee or school and preceptee)
- Identifies areas of concern in the preceptee's learning and provides additional help and teaching, either by themselves or by referring the preceptee to staff education or to the appropriate faculty member
- Consistently seeks out new learning opportunities for the preceptee, introducing them to new skills and opportunities

The ideal preceptor is a nurse who:

- Consistently role models evidence-based nursing practice and teaching how to prioritize patient care
- Documents and shares clinical progress and competence
- Never allows the preceptee to work above their scope of practice, and never allows others to ask this of the preceptee

The ideal preceptor is a leader and manager who:

- Teaches time management skills
- Consistently and constantly promotes problem-solving that utilizes critical reasoning and critical thinking
- Models effective communication skills when dealing with staff and patients
- Models effective conflict management skills
- Objectively assesses the preceptee's skills
- Provides constructive, not belittling, argumentative, or unsupportive feedback
- Values professional growth and encourage this in other nurses and staff members
- Takes time with the preceptee and acts to both nurture and coach

The ideal preceptor is an advocate for the preceptee who:

- Refers preceptee for unit and facility projects and committees
- Suggests opportunities for the preceptee to advance in their education and within their specialty
- Introduces the preceptee to members of the healthcare team and explains their role in the care of the patient and how they can be contacted
- Assists the preceptee in finding resources to answer their questions rather than automatically answering or finding the information for them
- Provides or shows the preceptee the location of key unit policies and procedure documents
- Accompanies the preceptee in all new tasks, skills, assessments, and experiences (never leaves the preceptee alone in a new situation)
- Completes all necessary paperwork and documentation regarding the successful (or unsuccessful) completion of the steps or preceptorship
- Encourages the preceptee to develop good self-care habits, such as taking meal breaks and getting sufficient rest
- Honestly discusses work-related stress, symptoms of burnout, compassion fatigue, and reality shock, how to deal with these issues, and provides sources of assistance

The ideal preceptor is a role model who:

- Has warmth
- Possess a sense of humor
- Is mature and self-confident
- Is able to handle success as well as failure
- Is empathetic to students, staff, and patients
- Is honest and accountable
- Has teaching as well as leadership skills
- Shows respect for fellow staff and the preceptees they work with
- Is enthusiastic about being a nurse and a preceptor

## BEING A MENTOR

Many mentors are preceptors, but not all preceptors are mentors, and that is unfortunate. *The Oxford English Dictionary* defines a mentor as "an experienced and trusted advisor." Isn't that what a nurse preceptor should be? To mentor another person is a form of fostering human development. The mentor invests time, energy, and passion into assisting another nurse in becoming what they were truly meant to be.

A mentor is, above all, a role model, not only to the preceptee but also to others in the profession. Mentors model the best of their profession in their interactions with others. A mentor is a respected and valuable resource not only to fellow nurses but also to many members of the healthcare team. So, knowing all this, shouldn't all preceptors be mentors?

Do you have what it takes to be a mentor to a nurse or student?

- Mentors are usually the most enthusiastic and "gung-ho" members of the team.
- They are the leaders; they desire to nurture a preceptee in their new role.
- They are the ones who think "outside the box" and will seek out situations in which to teach fellow team members.
- They actually embrace change rather than shying away from it and see change as a way to improve patient care rather than impede it.
- They don't just punch a clock or view their responsibilities as limited to their time at work. They work until they have completed a task or project.
- They don't hoard their knowledge but share it with others.
- Mentors are also fully aware that they don't have all the answers and are continually learning. They continually seek out situations in which the preceptee can grow both in skill level and experience.
- Mentors don't shield the preceptee from situations in which they may surpass them in experience and knowledge and aren't jealous; they cheer the preceptee on to excellence.
- Mentors exude empathy, knowledge, and patience for the preceptee, their patients, and fellow staff.
- Mentors are approachable and have good communication skills.
- Mentors have a strong sense of ethics. They incorporate ethical behavior into their teaching and communication in order to pass it on to other members of staff.
- They don't take themselves too seriously and have a good sense of humor.
- They show respect for other nurses, students, fellow staff, families, and patients.
- They are organized and dependable.

- They have excellent clinical skills.
- They have a varied background in nursing.
- They are realistic in their goals for the preceptee and in their own practice.
- They know and understand that they are shaping a preceptee's attitude about what constitutes excellence in nursing.

The key responsibilities of a preceptor who is a mentor include:

- Creating a welcoming environment for and working to develop a rapport with the preceptee
- Identifying the learning needs of the preceptee
- Organizing and coordinating the learning activities and ensuring that learned skills take place in practice
- Assisting the preceptee in meeting their stated goals
- Working in collaboration with staff education or faculty to set goals for the preceptee
- Supervising the preceptee in new learning situations
- Always acting in a professional and appropriate manner in any given situation; being a role model
- Providing patient care according to evidence-based nursing practice standards
- Following facility policy and procedures and ensuring that others do the same
- Working in collaboration with other members of the healthcare team
- Acting as a leader to other members of the team
- Taking pride in being a nurse, no matter the degree earned or specialty
- Sharing stories of success and offering helpful tips on how the preceptee can be successful

There are many ways in which a successful preceptor who is a mentor positively impacts the preceptee. A few examples follow.

- Preceptees or staff members feel comfortable asking questions, irrespective of whether they think their questions might be "silly." No one is belittled when they ask a question. The preceptor realizes that there are no "stupid" questions and never makes anyone feel as if they have asked one.
- Preceptees feel respected for what they can bring to a patient care situation, their interactions with fellow staff, and the learning environment as a whole.

- Preceptees are never made to feel uncomfortable or incompetent.
- Preceptees perceive that the mentor is able to empathize with them in their new role by being able to recall what it was like to be a new nurse, student, or employee. New or stressful situations are introduced by letting the preceptee know that the mentor was once in the same situation and understands.

## Characteristics of a Successful Mentor

The list of responsibilities and characteristics of a mentor is practically endless because being a mentor can mean different things to different people. It is clear, however, that mentors are committed professionals with a passion for nursing and a true interest in furthering the profession by giving of themselves. Once preceptorship is over and the preceptee has moved on, either as a student or in the role of staff nurse, the preceptor may take on the role of mentor. This should be considered when taking on the responsibility of preceptorship because your role in the life a preceptee extends past the end of the preceptorship.

Characteristics of a great mentor include the following:

- The mentor is an active listener. They don't assume to know the thoughts or feelings of others in any given situation but instead allow people time to express themselves in conversation.
- The mentor is consistent, and anyone working with them will know what is expected in their practice. Clinical and professional development goals are mutually agreed on, and they remain constant.
- The mentor shows a true desire to continually learn and to pass that love of learning on to others.
- The mentor continually challenges the preceptee to go beyond the expected, to continually question the norm and go further than current limits, and to envision the future of the profession.
- The mentor provides feedback based on objective observation of the progress (or lack thereof) of the preceptee.
- The mentor participates in continuing education activities and encourages others to do the same.
- The mentor assists with the growth of the preceptorship program by participating in ongoing evaluation and quality assurance.
- The mentor must also know that not all new nurses or students were meant to be nurses. They are not judgmental, or critical,

but understand that a person's skills, talents, and abilities may be suited to another area, practice, or profession and will point this out in a caring and understanding way. The mentor will also guide the preceptee to the specialty or profession for which the nurse may be better suited.

## PHASES OF PRECEPTORSHIP

As with any relationship, preceptorship involves phases through which the preceptor and preceptee move. There is not always a clear demarcation between the end of one phase and the beginning of another. Many goals and tasks are ongoing throughout the preceptorship period. But all preceptorships involve at least two main phases: (a) an establishment phase, in which the preceptorship relationship is initiated and trust is established, and (b) a working phase, in which the educational plan is established.

### Establishment Phase: Trust Is Established

In this phase, the preceptor:

- Seeks to provide a structured preceptorship, recognizing that anxiety felt by the preceptee may be decreased accordingly
- Creates a safe learning environment
- Provides an environment where the preceptee may learn from their mistakes in a non-punitive fashion
- Is open to the new ideas, information, or skills that the preceptee may bring to a situation. Avoid the "this is the way we've always done it" attitude
- Begins, prior to the commencement of orientation, with the review of employee/orientation documentation, including competency documentation

- Meets and assists faculty or staff education in the planning of the preceptorship process
- Encourages review of the preceptee's nursing skills through simulation prior to clinical placement, allowing the preceptor to assess the preceptee's preparedness for patient care
- Only allows the preceptee to perform care that is meaningful and with purpose; they are not on the unit to complete "busy" work or work that no one else wishes to perform
- Understands what the preceptee already knows and what they need to know
- Reviews with the preceptee their past clinical experiences, future career goals, and personal objectives; understands the preceptee's learning style and how it can be addressed with resources available within the facility
- Thoroughly outlines the orientation plan with the preceptee
- Orients the preceptee to the unit/facility and introduces them to fellow team members
- Discusses how often formal communication will occur (weekly or biweekly) and with whom, in addition to daily informal meetings
- Provides continuity in the first days of preceptorship, when roles are established and boundaries are outlined
- Provides feedback to the preceptee in determining their progress
- Encourages open and honest communication

### Working Phase: Implementation of the Education Plan

In this phrase, the preceptor:

- Acts above all as a role model for the preceptee, acting as consult and resource person
- Treats the preceptee with respect and dignity
- Never uses shame or humiliation as a "teaching tool"
- Shares their own clinical experiences thus providing the preceptee with a new insight and understanding of nursing and the preceptor
- Presents experiences in such a way as to develop critical thinking skills in the preceptee
- Models professional nursing skills as they apply to theory and science, problem-solving, and decision-making
- Encourages the preceptee to observe the preceptor and other staff as they care for patients and interact with other members of the healthcare team and families; discusses those interactions and observations with the preceptee

- Observes the professional skills of the nurse and provides regular feedback throughout this phase, including the preceptee's goals achievements
- Evaluates the preceptee's progress in learning and addresses any issues that are hindering learning
- Communicates regarding the care of patients, the feelings of the preceptee, and the recognition that ongoing learning is a daily occurrence
- Ensures that the preceptee is moving from a directed to a self-directed role, with the preceptee becoming more independent and the preceptor taking on a more observational role
- Ensures that goals are met or that goals are reestablished, reassessed, and reevaluated as needed
- Ensures that the preceptee is completing facility- or institution-required documentation such as daily logs or competency checklists, thus enabling both the preceptor and preceptee to visually track progress
- May feel a sense of loss as the preceptor–preceptee relationship progresses and changes (This is normal; the change can be discussed between the two, acknowledging its existence, but realizing they are moving forward.)
- Formally discusses any progress (or lack thereof) on the part of the preceptee with the appropriate institution or facility personnel, and documents as required
- Remembers that the goal of preceptorship is to either have a fully functioning staff member or successful student upon its completion. Preceptees are not to become dependent on the preceptor and no opportunity should be provided for this to occur.
- Apologizes when they are wrong, doesn't make promises they cannot keep, honors their commitments, is consistent in their words and actions, maintains their integrity, and maintains the highest level of patient care possible

## Fast Facts

One of the best ways to gain respect is to say, "I don't know" when asked a question by a preceptee that you truly don't know the answer to. You should not be reluctant to show that you don't have all the answers but be knowledgeable in how to find the answers

## References

Maguire, D. J., Zambroski, C. H., & Cadena, S. (2012). Using a clinical collaborative model for nursing education application for clinical teaching. *Nurse Educator, 37*(2), 80–85. doi:10.1097/NNE.0b013e3182461bb6

# 2

# Selection, Education, and Retention of the Preceptor

*Due to the continual decline in the number of nurse educators and the increasing need for capstone and preceptorship experiences, the need for well-educated, experienced, and willing preceptors has never been greater. Preceptors are key to staff retention, job satisfaction, continuing education, improved quality of care, patient safety, and transition to practice. We all know nurses who became preceptors because it was their "turn" to be one or they were assigned to be a preceptor by staff development. Being a preceptor may be a requirement that must be "checked off" on the way up a clinical ladder or for increased pay. Many nurses are not given the choice of becoming a preceptor, and this is unfortunate. Preceptors should receive proper education on how to be a preceptor in order to provide the best experience to the preceptee. Not every nurse can or should be a preceptor.*

After reading this chapter, the reader will be able to:

1. List the challenges facing a preceptor
2. List five qualities of a potential preceptor
3. List five benefits of a formal preceptor program
4. List five actions a facility can do to retain nurse preceptors

**5.** List five issues that lead to preceptor burnout

**6.** List the benefits that preceptors bring to a healthcare facility

## WHAT'S IN IT FOR YOU?

Being a preceptor is not easy! It often takes place in less than ideal conditions. For instance:

- The preceptor may have their own patient assignment while orienting a new nurse who also has a patient assignment, thus doubling the work (but not the compensation) of the preceptor.
- The preceptor may have to deal with unclear goals from the facility or school of nursing.
- There may be a lack of support from nursing administration and fellow staff.
- The preceptor may be unable to honestly evaluate a new nurse due to staffing pressures… "Hurry up and get this one trained so we can add them to the schedule."
- Preceptorship may result in a doubling of the amount of responsibility due to staffing pressures and decreasing patient safety.

Preceptors may not be compensated for their time as a preceptor. They may be chosen because they are "next in line" to be used to orient new staff and may not have received education in precepting. The institution may not value the preceptorship concept and may utilize a new nurse as staff before orientation has ended, or may not offer a comprehensive preceptorship program from the start. Perhaps, after reading this text and understanding how your facility supports (or does not support) the preceptorship model, you will feel empowered to begin the process of advocating that preceptors become valued by the facility, nursing management, and fellow staff at your facility.

What benefit does preceptorship have for both the preceptor and the preceptee? The rewards for the nursing staff, facility, and patients are many, such as:

- Learning new skills
- Improving current patient care skills
- Ensuring that excellent, safe care is provided by future nurses
- Increased job and career satisfaction
- Increased self-esteem and feeling of confidence
- Increased influence on facility nursing practice

- Professional development
- Development of teaching skills
- Improvement of leadership skills
- Helping the preceptor realize their dreams
- The preceptee growing in skill and confidence, and utilizing evidence-based practice experienced in preceptorship
- Decrease in staff turnover

### Fast Facts

Many nurses become preceptors and educators because of their experiences in orientation or preceptorship. They either wish to share the experience they had or make sure a negative experience is not perpetuated.

## SELECTION OF A NURSE PRECEPTOR

To provide the best preceptorship experience for the student or new nurse and the highest patient quality care and safety, understand how a preceptor *should be* selected from your nursing staff. If you were to ask a nurse educator what type of nurse makes the best preceptor, they would probably list the following attributes:

- Sound clinical skills
- Team player
- Capacity to think critically and use problem-solving skills effectively
- Ability to effectively communicate with fellow healthcare providers, patients, and families
- Positive attitude
- Positive role model
- Strong desire to teach
- Excellent teaching ability
- Sensitive to the learning needs of students and new nurses
- Clear desire to grow professionally; constantly seeking new educational opportunities
- Strong leadership abilities
- Contributes to the clinical skills of the unit/facility
- Objectivity

- Practices with compassionate care
- Available to assist students and new nurses in completing projects or meeting objectives
- Participates in community and facility committees that further the practice of nursing or regarding the improvement of healthcare

Not every nurse has these skills or has them in differing quantities, and a nurse should not be selected to be a preceptor just based on their clinical skills alone. So how does a nurse educator, faculty member, or nurse manager know which nurse would make the best preceptor? Obviously, only those nurses who express an interest in precepting should be chosen. Hospitals who possess or who are seeking ANCC (American Nurses Credentialing Center) Magnet status should select preceptors who exemplify the values of the ANCC. The ANCC standards, however, exemplify the ideal nurse and should be utilized by all facilities developing a preceptor program to ensure that the best candidates are selected.

The ANCC acknowledges there are factors central to furthering the profession of nursing, reforming the healthcare system, and improving the care of the patient, family, and community. They utilize the phrase "Global Issues in Nursing and Health Care" and within its foundation lay the issues facing nursing and healthcare, such as new knowledge, innovation, and improvements; exemplary professional practice; and empirical quality outcomes, structural empowerment, and transformational leadership. Within each of these is a "forces of magnetism," the history of which goes back to the founding of Magnet research in the 1980s. Elizabeth Cotter, PhD, RN-BC PhD, RN-BC, in her 2016 article "Professional Development of Preceptors Improves Nurse Outcomes" noted that a preceptor candidate should exemplify these forces (Table 2.1).

## Table 2.1

### Preceptor Candidate Forces

| The Quality of Nursing Leadership | Patient and Staff Advocate |
| --- | --- |
| Organizational Structure | Represents nursing on different facility committees and participates in shared decision-making that affects the organization as a whole. |

(continued)

## Table 2.1

### Preceptor Candidate Forces (*continued*)

| The Quality of Nursing Leadership | Patient and Staff Advocate |
| --- | --- |
| Management Style | Assists in creating a supportive working environment where constructive feedback is encouraged, appreciated, and assimilated into care. Nurses in positions of leadership are accessible to all staff and model effective communication. |
| Personnel Policies and Programs | Supports and encourages professional growth and education among fellow nurses. Participates in the development of policies and procedures that support professional nursing practice and improvement in patient quality care. |
| Professional Models of Care | Encourages administration to support models of nursing care that give the nursing staff direct responsibility and authority for patient care (coordination of care) such as primary nursing and case management. |
| Quality of Care | Supports an environment where quality care is the driving force behind all of the actions of the facility. It should be understood by all nurses that they are to provide high-quality care to all of their patients. |
| Quality Improvement | Participates in quality improvement processes. |
| Consultation and Resources | Participates in professional organizations and outside community organizations. Supports the use of advanced practice nurses within the facility. |
| Autonomy | Provides competent, professional, knowledgeable nursing care that is evidence based and consistent with professional standards. After seeking the input of nursing and other care disciplines, correctly utilizes independent judgment as to what patient care should be provided. |
| Community and Healthcare Organization | Promotes and participates in healthcare and community organizations in order to promote improved healthcare outcomes. |

(*continued*)

## Table 2.1

### Preceptor Candidate Forces (*continued*)

| The Quality of Nursing Leadership | Patient and Staff Advocate |
| --- | --- |
| Nurses as Teachers | Involved in educational activities within the facility and also in the outside community. Welcomes and supports all levels of students. Participates in the development and/or ongoing success of a mentoring program for all preceptors. |
| Image of Nursing | Promotes nursing as an integral and valued member of the healthcare team. Nurses are influential in facility-wide patient care services. |
| Interdisciplinary Relationships | Values the working relationships among all facility healthcare disciplines. Promotes mutual respect and expresses that all members of the healthcare team provide meaningful contributions to patient care. Effectively utilizes conflict management. |
| Professional Development | Promotes the professional growth of ALL members of the healthcare team, not just nursing staff, including attaining of higher degrees and professional certifications. Assists in the development of competency-based clinical and leadership programs. |

Obviously, the staff who works with the proposed preceptor and the educators who have observed them should also have input as to who becomes a preceptor. Only nurses who have received positive evaluations from their peers and managers should be among those selected. The literature further states that in addition to strong clinical skills with up-to-date clinical competency measurement, cultural sensitivity, good interpersonal skills, excellent communication skills, enthusiasm about nursing, independent thinking, participation in facility and community groups that further the profession of nursing or improve healthcare, knowledge of unit and facility policies and procedures, a model of excellent nursing care and practice, positive outlook, organized, adaptable, learner empathy, and strong desire to teach, potential preceptors should also possess a BSN or higher degree, and be a full-time employee with a minimum of three years' work experience as an RN. The patient care skills of the nurse should be observed by a nurse educator to ensure that they meet the clinical competencies of the chosen specialty unit.

If only there was a tool that could assist in the decision-making process! Such an instrument would eliminate subjectivity and be consistently accurate and reliable. Unfortunately, very little research has been conducted on how to recognize, choose, and assess a preceptor, so no one tool exists. Any tool used must address the needs and concerns of the American Nurses Association Nursing: Scope and Standards of Practice and be exclusive to nursing (not adapted from another profession).

Cotter and her colleagues developed and tested a preceptor selection instrument in 2015. This instrument was "developed using the American Nurses Association Nursing: Scope and Standards of Practice...it was created based on a literature review of positive preceptor attributes...it addressed the areas of clinical competence, nursing process, transformational leadership, collaboration/communication, professional development, conflict resolution, commitment, flexibility, empowerment and values...It uses a 3 point Likert scale ranging from 1 = needs improvement, 2 = meets expectations to 3 = exceeds expectations. A total score of 35 or greater is required for a nurse to be eligible to become a preceptor" (Cotter, Eckardt, & Moylan, 2018). After a study on a small sample, Cotter noted the instrument was valid and could be used to aid in preceptor selection. She recommends further testing of the instrument within larger and more diverse nursing populations but feels that it can be used as an accepted rating system for preceptor selection.

There are traits commonly accepted as being the primary roles of a preceptor. They include:

- Role model
- Teacher
- Coach or nurturer
- Professional resource
- Socializer
- Observer
- Evaluator
- Organizer

## EDUCATION OF A NURSE PRECEPTOR

Being a preceptor is challenging. It is more so especially if the preceptor has not been properly educated to their role and lacks support. Challenges faced by the preceptor could be:

- Time constraints
- No communication between preceptor and faculty or staff development
- No interaction among fellow preceptors for shared experiences and learning
- Lack of a formal preceptorship structure
- Lack of policies, procedures, and protocols governing preceptorship
- Poor to no compensation
- No education to the role
- Lack of appreciation and support

A formal preceptor development program not only educates *how* to be a preceptor but it also provides a network of support and collaboration. Policies, procedures, and protocols provide role clarity and a clear understanding of the expectations of the preceptor experience. The critical thinking ability of the preceptor is enriched, which, in turn, assists in developing increased critical reasoning in the preceptee. Unfortunately, again, there is not much in the literature regarding the development of a preceptor program. But because of decreased availability of faculty, strong competition for clinical sites (and a decrease in their availability), and an increase in the number of nurses entering the profession at different levels (BSN, DNP, NP, etc.), it is vital that preceptor programs are in place.

The first step is to ensure facility "buy-in." Meet with administration, unit managers, clinical specialists, current preceptors, clinical educators, facility nurse educators, and faculty from colleges/universities utilizing your facility as a clinical area. Delineate for them what the preceptor program would contain, the curriculum, policies, goals, and expected outcomes and benefits. Be sure to list the benefits to the facility (i.e., job satisfaction, decreased staff turnover, better patient outcomes, better quality of care, increased patient safety, etc.). All participants need to fully support and value the program for it to succeed. Emphasize that significant communication and responsibility must take place among all the partners (administration, educators, faculty members, nursing staff, preceptors, and preceptees) for the program to meet its outcomes and be successful.

A preceptor program should have clear policies that denote the following:

- How nursing administrators, staff development educators, and nursing faculty identify who may be a nursing preceptor
- Once chosen among their peers, how the preceptor is selected to continue on with preceptor education (standardized testing)
- Clarification of the role of the preceptor
- Compensation for preceptor
- Expectations of the preceptor

## CURRICULUM OF A PRECEPTOR PROGRAM

Preceptor development programs differ in offered curriculum and how that curriculum is delivered. It is recommended, however, that due to staffing constraints, if a preceptor is removed from the staffing schedule for an extended period, then the facility should consider online learning as well as classroom and skills lab. Currently, some nursing specialties have preceptor courses available online (links available in the resources section).

Common elements of a preceptor curriculum:

- Review of facility patient care policies and procedures
- Review of roles and responsibilities of all involved
- Review of program goals and expected outcomes (should be measurable)
- Creation of a safe and positive learning environment
- Adult learning principles
- Conflict resolution
- Cultural diversity
- Delegation
- Skills review
- How to provide feedback (constructive and positive)
- Prioritization
- Time management
- Review and understanding of any documentation related to orientation and preceptorship
- Record keeping of documents utilized for orientation/ preceptorship
- Effective preceptee assessment and evaluation

- Evidence-based practice and utilizing research
- Critical thinking, clinical judgment, clinical reasoning
- Quality improvement
- Clinical resources, where to find and how to use
- Teaching skills and styles
- Working with the competencies of specific units
- Organizing the clinical day
- What to communicate with administration and nursing education (progress of the preceptee, issues of concern, recommendations, changes/improvements, meeting of unit specific benchmarks)
- Review of job descriptions
- Orientation and onboarding

At the end of the program, those attending should complete an evaluation to ascertain what about the program was/was not beneficial and what subjects should be added or modified. An informal study should also be conducted to determine whether a greater number of nursing staff were retained and if this number demonstrated an improvement. Note other benefits of the program and report these to all facility parties.

## RETENTION OF THE PRECEPTOR

Burnout of the preceptor does occur, not only because of the stresses of nursing but also because of the increased stress of also being a preceptor. Burnout develops due to:

- Increased responsibility
- Inability to complete a patient care assignment to their level of satisfaction due to increased workload
- Increased patient workload due to preceptor/preceptee assignment
- High patient acuity (may be increased due to teaching needs of the preceptee)
- Lack of administrative support
- No formal preceptor education
- No formal preceptor program
- Facility and nursing staff attitude that the preceptee is just the preceptors "helper"
- Nursing administration utilizing preceptee as staff prior to end of preceptorship
- Ill-prepared nursing students or new staff nurses
- Lack of appreciation, recognition, and compensation

## Fast Facts

When asked, many preceptors stated that being a preceptor is its own reward. That the gratitude of the preceptee and the knowledge that they assisted in the development of an excellent nurse was recognition enough.

Monetary compensation would be wonderful for the preceptor. Unfortunately, not many facilities provide this benefit. There are other ways to assist in the retention of the preceptor and they include:

- Creation of a formal preceptor program
- Provide for networking opportunities among the preceptors in the facility
- Provide mentors for the preceptors; provide opportunities for preceptor interaction
- Nursing and facility administration support and full buy-in to the preceptor process
- Recognize that the preceptor/preceptee team is not on the unit to take on more patients and decrease the patient load of other nursing staff
- Provide tuition reimbursement for preceptors seeking an advanced degree and or continuing education
- Provide opportunities for the preceptor to attend continuing education courses
- Pay increase during preceptor period or bonus pay
- Contact hours for preceptor and other courses completed
- Provide for formal meeting times for facility preceptors to meet as a group for support and exchange of ideas. Provide time for the preceptors to leave the unit to attend the meetings or compensate for days off
- Show formal appreciation recognized by the facility such as gifts or luncheons. Include their contribution to nursing with articles in facility-wide newsletters
- Honor preceptors with special awards, perhaps noting their contributions during Nurses Week
- Participate in regularly scheduled meetings among administration, managers, preceptors, and educators to discuss the progress of the preceptees. Do not cancel these meetings as it shows a lack of concern and respect.

# MYERS BRIGGS PERSONALITY ASSESSMENT

Some schools of nursing utilize the Myers Briggs Type Indicator® (MBTI®) to match preceptors with preceptees. You can read more about at the link provided in the Resources section.

They have found that it is easier to work with someone of your same personality than a randomly selected individual. Potential preceptors can be tested prior to the start of preceptorship as can preceptees. If the school or facility has a pool of preceptors that have undergone training in a preceptorship program, they could undergo the testing and be available for when a "match" is ready.

The MBTI® personality inventory brings order to what seems like random personality traits and behavior. It is based on how individuals perceive and judge their surroundings and interactions with others. It can be concluded that if a person reacts and judges things differently they will also differ in what they value, what skills they possess, what motivates them, and what interests them (MBTI, 2020).

## Resources

### Online Preceptor Courses

https://www.aacn.org/education/online-courses/the-preceptor-challenge
http://www.preceptoracademy.com/
https://kchealthcareers.com/
http://lippincottsolutions.lww.com/solutions/development/collection.html
http://vchclinicaleducation.ca/wp-content/uploads/2017/03/Preceptorship
-Manual-Print-2007-dec.pdf

## References

Cotter, E., Eckardt, P., & Moylan, L. (2018). Instrument development and testing for selection of nursing preceptors. *Journal for Nurses in Professional Development. 34*(4), 185–193. doi:10.1097/NND.0000000000000464

The Myers and Briggs Foundation. (2020). *Take the MBTI instrument.* Retrieved from https://www.myersbriggs.org/my-mbti-personality-type/take-the-mbti-instrument/home.htm?bhcp=1

# 3

# Preceptee Learning and Preceptor Teaching Styles

*"Everyone learns differently." All educators have heard that in their career, but what exactly does that mean? How do teaching/ learning styles translate in the clinical area? How does someone who may have never formally taught before (i.e., your typical nursing preceptor) teach a preceptee? All preceptors, as part of their responsibilities, should take the time to ascertain how their preceptee learns. All preceptors should be able to teach with different styles depending on how their preceptee best learns. You are not expected to be an educational expert, but you can learn about different teaching strategies to assist your preceptee. A nurse's attitude toward teaching is very often formed by how they were taught. We vow that if "we ever precept we will never _____," or we state "if we ever get to teach we will remember to _____." We witness the outcome of how nurses were taught as we work beside them in various clinical settings.*

After reading this chapter, the reader will be able to:

1. List five principles of adult learning
2. Describe the types of learners
3. Describe the three domains of learning
4. Describe five teaching strategies for a novice learner
5. List the stages of competence

All learning takes places on a continual basis and learning styles will differ from one preceptee to another. All preceptees come "pre-equipped" to the clinical area with:

- Personal history
- Information on various subjects
- Values, beliefs, and opinions
- "Baggage" from how they were treated by educators/past preceptors
- Personal learning style
- The ability to relate new information to what was learned in the past

For every preceptee the preceptor encounters, they should:

- Ask the preceptee prior to the start of preceptorship how they learn and what method(s) work best for them. The preceptor can briefly assess the learning style of the preceptee by asking, "Do you learn better by reading, by listening, by observing, through hands-on activities, or a combination of these?" You can also utilize the self-tests found in the Resources section.
- Allow the preceptee to learn at their own pace, without rushing them and without showing impatience. All members of the healthcare team who interact with and teach your preceptee should also use the same methods of teaching.
- Allow the preceptee to test their own ideas or theories, review and learn from mistakes, be creative, and encourage "out-of-the-box" thinking. All of these will help to build critical thinking skills.
- It is acceptable to use different teaching methods to address a learning need.
- If you are finding that one method is not working, communicate with the preceptee and test a different method. Remember to speak to faculty who may have some insight as well. Involve the preceptee in reviewing different learning methods that they think will assist them.

**Fast Facts**

"We remember 10% of what we read, 20% of what we hear, 30% of what we see, 50% of what we see and hear, 70% of what we discuss with others, 80% of what we personally experience and 95% of what we teach others" (Learning & Career Development, Vancouver Coastal Health, 2006).

# ADULT LEARNING

There are various principles of adult learning. Some references list between five to 10, and the summation of them are listed here:

1.  Adults learn by doing. aAsk the preceptee to demonstrate a new skill. Do not show impatience if this demonstration is slow or mistakes are made. If working with a patient and not in simulation, be sure the preceptee is safely performing the skill.

2.  Adults learn by focusing on one task at a time. Teach one concept or skill before moving to another.

3.  Adults must be mentally and physically ready to learn. Assess if the preceptee is ready to learn a new concept or skill. Are they stressed or anxious? Assist them in dealing with any distractions before attempting education.

4.  Adults must be motivated to learn. Assess what motivates the preceptee. Are they nearing graduation? What makes them want to succeed and become a nurse?

5.  Material taught to the preceptee must be meaningful to them. Preceptors and educators should focus on what is needed, with no extraneous information… "How does what I'm teaching relate to the care of the patient?" Preceptees will focus on information that is the most useful to them.

6.  Adults who use critical thinking (though this skill must be learned further), ask "why" and "why not" questions and assess the reliability of information. They seek patterns and themes in information.

7.  Adults learn from exercises that are as real as possible, such as case studies and simulations.

8.  Educators should connect previously learned information and accumulated life experiences with new knowledge. The preceptor should respect the experiences that the preceptee brings to their patient care and connect new learning to it.

9.  Adults require immediate feedback after demonstrating what they have learned. Feedback must be consistent and constructive (see Chapter 8, The Value of Feedback).

10. Adult response to learning varies. Preceptors should be aware of the preceptees perception of their learning. Do they feel they are learning?

11. Adult learners are usually self-directed. Not only should goals that need to be achieved during preceptorship be set for them by faculty or the preceptor, the preceptee should also actively develop their own goals and ways to achieve them with preceptor guidance.

12. The learning environment can stimulate or adversely impact learning.Ensure that the learning environment you create is safe and allows the preceptee to make mistakes without humiliation or embarrassment. The trust bond you have with the preceptee should begin on the first day of preceptorship(see Chapter 1, Preceptorship in a Nutshell).

13. Adults are goal-oriented. They usually are aware of what they want to learn and they must have a reason for learning. They may have an issue with learning things in sequence or "the little things" so share with them the "big picture" and the end results in what they are learning.

14. The background and physical abilities of the preceptee will vary. Learn what they value, what they consider a challenge, and their strengths.

## TYPES OF LEARNERS

To understand how others learn, first understand how *you* learn. Select one or more of the quizzes found in the Resources section.

There are three main types of learners: visual, auditory, and kinesthetic. Learners can also be a combination of these types as well.

- The Visual Learner—learns by visual activity
  - Provide visual study materials, such as videos, notes, charts, or flashcards
  - Advise them to practice visualizing what they are learning in their head
  - Advise them to write out their class notes for review
    - Preceptor Hint: Allow the preceptee to read about a skill prior to performing. Let them review policies and procedures to understand them rather than just telling them what they are.
- The Auditory Learner—learns by hearing
  - Should tape lectures or presentations
  - Should sit close to the instructor
  - Summarize notes and read them aloud
    - Preceptor Hint: Discuss the skill to be performed or read the policy and procedure out loud to them.
- The Kinesthetic Learner—learns by hands-on activity
  - Uses sense of touch to assist in learning
  - Advise them to write notes or key facts several times over
  - Learns best from simulation

❏   Preceptor Hint: Allow the preceptee to learn by doing.
    Allow them to perform a skill in order to fully understand
    what it entails.

The acquisition of knowledge takes place on three different levels
or domains within the mind. The three domains of learning are
described in Table 3.1. For a more in-depth review, follow the link in
the Resources section.

Table 3.1

## The Three Domains of Learning

| Domain | Affective | Cognitive | Psychomotor |
|---|---|---|---|
| Definition | Behavioral, beliefs, values | Knowledge-based | Skill-based |
| What it means for the preceptee | The preceptee can display, exhibit, and accept. The preceptee is able to require the necessary knowledge and then distinguish when that knowledge should be used in the care of the patient. | The preceptee understands facts (concepts), puts two or more of them together (to compare, to contrast, to describe), and can then apply them (explain, apply, or analyze). | The preceptee can demonstrate, at the bedside, what they have learned. |
| What it means for preceptor | To teach to this domain, use discussion, and to test knowledge, observe the preceptee and their interactions with the patient. | To teach to this domain, speak directly to the preceptee and use written materials. To test their knowledge, utilize debriefing sessions or case studies | To teach this domain, allow the preceptee to imitate your actions (return demonstration) and provide time for practice (once competent, without preceptor monitoring); eventually the preceptee will develop the skill into a habit. To test their knowledge, use skill testing. |

## Preceptees Are Novices Too

When precepting, always remember what it was like when you were beginning your career. Remember what it was like to be a student in clinical, a graduate nurse in preceptorship, or a new nursing employee. The accelerated student or new nurse may have been an expert in their prior jobs and are now starting over again in a new profession. Never assume a preceptee who is doing well does not require strong preceptor support. As the preceptee progresses in skill development, make sure that their patient acuity increases as well.

As previously stated, limit their strict observations of you or other healthcare workers performing care. While observation is fine, it should not become a major part of their preceptorship. It should be used to demonstrate a skill or interaction once or twice or as requested by the preceptee or as needed by the preceptor. Consider learning outside of the clinical area. Hear a code called? How about that rapid response on another unit? Let the preceptee observe the action and discuss their observations with you.

## "I Don't Know!"

The preceptor should always be prepared for the question they can't answer! Many preceptors live in fear of this and really they should not. You are not expected to know everything, and you shouldn't feel that you should.

Another fear that preceptors have is that "a new skill has been developed or a new way to do what I've always done has been proposed and I'm going to look stupid!" Never be afraid to say that you do not know something. Never say "I don't know" and leave it at that either! Use this opportunity for what it is...a learning opportunity. You will show that nurses should never stop learning. Be aware of resources for your unit and the facility so if you ARE asked a question you don't know the answer to, you can research the answer and assist the preceptee to do the same.

## NOVICE LEARNERS

- Nervous, anxious, lacking in self-confidence with no immediate emotional support in their new environment
- So focused on the task at hand they may miss important patient information which interferes with assessment, problem anticipation, and prioritization

- May be unable to multi-task
- Anxiety may be at such a level at the beginning of preceptorship that it may be more beneficial for the preceptor to tell the preceptee what to do rather than questioning to build critical thinking skills
- Monitor the preceptee and encourage them to focus on learning new skills and not become distracted

Clinical teaching strategies for a novice learner:

- As stated previously, create a positive learning environment that will help to decrease stress.
- Have empathy and remember what it was like to first begin your clinical experiences. But remember that your preceptee may be a novice at nursing but an expert in something else, or may not be sufficient in one skill but proficient in others.
- Identify and acknowledge the preceptee's strengths and remind them of those strengths because they may be so stressed they forget!
- Help them to identify and verbalize what they may be afraid of... work to eliminate that fear.
    - For example, many preceptees are afraid the preceptor will leave them alone with a new skill...so don't! Always be with the preceptee when they perform a new skill (or when they ask for you to be present to help ease their anxiety at any time). As their anxiety lessens and their skills improve, you can move from closely monitoring them to checking in on them as needed.
- Avoid information overload at the beginning of preceptorship. Give simple, clear instructions. You will then move forward from this to the questions preparing them to think critically.
- Move from simple to more complex information and remember to focus only on relevant information.
- Build new information on what the preceptee already knows.
- Break major skills down into smaller, more manageable parts and present the task in that way. For example: If you are inserting a urinary catheter you may list each step as a separate task (patient assessment, washing hands, patient positioning, setting up the sterile field) etc.
- Expect to repeat information but do so in a non-hurried, non-judgmental way, understanding that repetition helps with the learning process.
- Encourage the preceptee to ask questions, reassure them there are no "stupid questions."

- If they are showing their anxiety, assure them that it is normal to be nervous and do what you can to decrease the anxiety (remove them from a situation, decrease the amount of information you are trying to provide).

## THE STAGES OF COMPETENCE

Also known as the four stages of learning, the preceptee should move through several states of competence during their time with the preceptor. They will also enter the clinical area, whether for school or starting a new job, at different stages and not necessarily the beginning. It is important to know what stage the preceptee is in when you first approach them so you can adjust your teaching style and then acknowledge the progression with adjusting your style again.

### Unconscious Incompetence

The preceptee does not know what they do not know. In other words, they don't know what skills they lack and what information they don't possess.

- Ask the preceptee what they plan to do for their care of the patient.
- Have the preceptee return demonstrate any skill with you.
- Help the preceptee to set realistic learning goals.
- Guide them without being negative about what they may be able to or not be able to do at this stage of learning.
- Learning may not take place at this stage.

### Conscious Incompetence

Having now realized what they don't know, they discover that what they want to do may not be easy but they acknowledge the importance of learning something new.

- Verbalize your support of the preceptee. Let them know that one day they will "get it."
- If they are nervous about trying a new skill, remind them of your full support.
- Break down new skills into stages and progress towards the complex.
- Learning takes place at this stage.

## Conscious Competence

The preceptee is now competent in a skill, but focuses on the skill rather than the skill AND the patient because the skill requires active concentration; it is not performed automatically.

- Assist the preceptee by allowing them time to mentally or physically rehearse the skill in simulation.
- Don't distract them while they are performing the skill unless they are about to make a mistake or harm the patient.
- Engage the patient in conversation while the preceptee is performing a skill (if acceptable). In this way, the preceptee is not trying to talk to the patient and perform the task at the same time.
- Once the preceptee is competent and you have observed them, you may allow them to perform the skill on their own if they feel comfortable (but always acknowledge your availability for support).

## Unconsciously Competent

At this stage, the skill is now automatic and does not require conscious thinking. This step comes with extensive experience—the preceptee may not reach this stage while with the preceptor, but the preceptor exists at this stage. Therefore, there are alterations in your practice you can make to assist the preceptee with learning.

- Review the steps of a procedure so you can explain them to the preceptee. Review the rationale for what you are doing so that you can explain them as well.
- Speak the steps you are doing out loud while you are doing them with the preceptee. Be prepared to explain what, how, and why you are doing something.
- If appropriate, explain to the patient the steps you are taking while performing a skill. It will help to educate both preceptee AND the patient. If the information is not appropriate for the patient, be sure to share it with the preceptee in private at a later time.
- With any skill, there is a wrong way and a correct way to complete it. Every nurse may have a different method of performing the same task. As long as it is safe, follows evidence-based methods, is ethical, and works, it is okay. All nurses, including your preceptee, will find their own way to complete a skill or task. They must be

able to verbalize to you the rationale for why they are performing the skill the way they are and it must meet the above criteria.

■ Be a role model but always remember how you felt when you learned a new task.

■ The preceptor should always be prepared for the question they can't answer! Many preceptors live in fear of this and really they should not.

## HOW THE GENERATIONS LEARN

The difference among the generations has been reviewed in previous studies. For the purposes of this text, know the differences because all nurses must interact with other professionals from many different generations. Because of the life experiences of different generations, we can learn from each other and develop different ways of thinking and understanding, which leads to better teamwork and job satisfaction and safe patient outcomes. These are generalities and may vary among people. Very often, a lack of understanding of the values of others leads to conflict and a lack of appreciation. The following lists the generational differences and how it affects nursing:

■ Veterans (1925–1945)—Believe in the value of work, value sacrificing for the common good, have a longterm loyalty to an institution, respect authority, look to the past for what has worked, and may be technologically challenged.

■ Baby Boomers (1946–1964)—Now represent two-thirds of all workers in the United States and many are retiring from nursing, leaving a shortage in their wake. Have a strong work ethic. They expect to be able to freely express themselves and want to make an impact on their careers and the lives of their patients. Became nurses when the industry was MD order-driven rather than being independent in the patient care decisions. They are valued coaches and mentors.

■ Generation X (1965–1980)—They are loyal to their nursing career but not to the point of sacrificing their personal and family life. They seek positions where they have more control over their work schedule. They are usually tech-savvy and are valued for this. They are skilled in developing innovative processes for patient care. They are valued for their unique ideas and creativity and they assist healthcare facilities with developing new approaches to patient care.

- Generation Y (1980–2000)—This generation of nurses is usually ambitious and demanding. They request and require feedback and praise. Preceptor and mentor support is imperative to retain the novice nurse. They can work with the input of large amounts of data from different sources and have little tolerance for inefficiency and ineffectiveness. They are team players, sociable, and optimistic. They utilize their technical skills to develop innovative processes to produce cost-effective patient outcomes. Unfortunately, they have had little instruction on how to prioritize their patient care due to a limited amount of clinical sites, a lack of nurse educators, and a lack of opportunity to care for more than one patient during their clinical rotations. They may require assistance from a preceptor or mentor in following the hierarchy of leadership in a facility because they do not value leadership as past generations have. They will achieve more at a younger age, manifesting in younger nurses attending graduate school.

- Generation Z (2000 to present)—"Little is known about Gen Z nursing students… How many Gen Zers will enter nursing is uncertain. Much Gen Z research is marketing data because they comprise 40% of the consumer sector; research about career choices is still emerging. Given their characteristic strong work ethic, cautious nature, self-fulfillment over salary (altruism), and job stability, there is reason to suspect Gen Z students may pursue nursing… Keeping Gen Z students engaged will be a feat for nursing faculty. Gen Z students' attention spans are an astonishing 8 seconds, 4 seconds less than Millennials. Gen Zers learn by observation and practice. They do not want lecture and prefer doing over memorizing. Gen Zers learn by solving real-world problems. Gen Z students do not engage in long conversations, communicating instead in short bits and pieces. Their preferred communication method is texting, Twitter, and Snapchat. Gen Z students want to collaborate often, thinking independently at first and then discussing as a group. If they have questions, they will find the answers on YouTube and move on." (Williams, 2019)

## Fast Facts

"Tell them what you are going to tell them, tell them, then tell them what you told them." Aristotle

## Resources

### Learning Style Assessments

http://www.educationplanner.org/students/self-assessments/learning-styles
-quiz.shtml

http://www.whatismylearningstyle.com/learning-style-test-1.html

## References

Learning & Career Development, Vancouver Coastal Health. (2006). *Preceptor resource guide: Supporting clinical learning.* Retrieved from https://static1.squarespace.com/static/555cfb18e4b039100196660b/t/55949d65e4b0c83b49257bfc/1435802981934/Preceptor+Resource+Guide-Supporting+Clinical+Learning.pdf

Williams, C. (2019). Nurse educators meet your new students: Generation Z. *Nurse Educator, 44*(2), 59–60. doi:10.1097/NNE.0000000000000637

## Bibliography

Education Planner.org. (n.d.). *What's your learning style*? Retrieved from http://www.educationplanner.org/students/self-assessments/learning-styles-quiz.shtml

Explorable. (n.d.). *Domains of learning.* Retrieved from https://explorable.com/domains-of-learning

Training Industry. (2017). *The stages of competence.* Retrieved from https://trainingindustry.com/wiki/strategy-alignment-and-planning/the-four-stages-of-competence/

University of California – Irvine Medical Center. (2011). *Principles of adult learning and learning style assessment.* Irvine, CA: Department of Nursing Quality, Research and Education.

VARK. (n.d.). *The VARK questionnaire.* Retrieved from https://vark-learn.com/the-vark-questionnaire/

# 4

# The Challenging Student

*Students who are considered a challenge to preceptors fall into two main characteristics; those with learning problems and those with attitudinal issues (Hendricson & Kleffner, 2002).*

*Those with learning problems display performance issues consistently below the expectations of a nursing student or new nurse. Beware of when a preceptee who was performing at or above expectations suddenly develops a learning issue, as this may be a sign of something other than a learning problem. The preceptee with an attitudinal issue may continually frustrate the preceptor, be an unsafe practitioner, and be disruptive to others in the clinical area. Again, be aware of behavior changes in your preceptee as they can be a manifestation of medical conditions or drug/alcohol dependency.*

After reading this chapter, the reader will:

1. List the three most common types of altitudinal behavior
2. List six factors related to learning difficulties
3. List three issues that may interfere with preceptor learning
4. List three signs of an undiagnosed learning disability
5. Describe the use of PRIME in teaching

## PRECEPTEE BEHAVIOR

**Fast Facts**

The three common types of attitudinal behavior observed in preceptees are "acute defensiveness" which blocks communication between preceptee and preceptor, "lack of personal motivation" and "the know it all" (Hendricson & Kleffner, 2002).

All of these manifestations are thought to be defense mechanisms used to cover their fear and lack of knowledge and the hope that they can fake their way through to completion of preceptorship or graduation.

There are six factors related to learning difficulties. They can be seen in isolation or in combination.

- **Cognition**—This is related to how a preceptee acquires, processes, stores, and retrieves information (Hendricson & Kleffner, 2002). This is seen in the clinical area in preceptees due to poor curriculum format, the teaching methods of past clinical instructors or faculty, or how the preceptee studies. Because they were taught or study so poorly, the preceptee cannot retrieve information. They are unable to answer questions designed to help them think critically or verbalize the anticipated care of the patient. They cannot think "on the fly" as to what to anticipate in their care of the patient or what actions to take if any unexpected patient issues occur.
- **Study Habits**—If a preceptee has not learned to study, they are unable to learn.
- **Quality of the Academic Environment**—Learning is difficult when the curriculum is poorly formulated and implemented.
- **Student Distraction**—Preceptees, especially those in accelerated programs, have "life distractions" that can contribute to high stress levels and poor academic performance.
- **Affective Components**—As preceptees move through nursing school or their new job, the relationship they have with their educators evolves. The educator or preceptor may at one point be seen as hindering the preceptee's progress toward graduation, as helping them move through nursing school, or as the enemy or a friend. All of this affects learning.

- **Underlying medical problems**—Usually when all other causes of learning issues have been ruled out, consider that the preceptee faces chronic stress, may have previous medical issues or newly diagnosed medical issues, or may be dealing with chemical or another dependency,all of which affects memory and cognition and can lead to lack of attention, lack of energy, and emotional distress.

So what happens if preceptee learning is not affected by any of these six factors? Preceptors should then ask themselves the following questions:

## Is the Preceptee Unable to Retrieve Information?

The difference between a novice and an expert is how they are able to retrieve previously learned information. Healthcare workers must take information learned from lectures and books, verbalize the information in their own words, and link it to a current patient situation. A novice struggles with this, and an expert is able to instantly retrieve the information and solve a problem. A student who is unable to do this or who is still in the novice stage may exhibit the following characteristics:

- Long responses to answers that never address the question
- Inability to analyze data such as lab work and recognize patterns
- Inability to discuss a patient's care in-depth, unable to discuss what may be causing a disease process or symptoms
- Inability to explain how drugs interact with the patient's condition and the effect on body systems.
- Inability to explain the difference in disease processes (i.e., differing anemias or conditions of shock)
- Displays "anchoring" (Hendricson & Kleffner, 2002) in which the preceptee is unable to change their opinion on the care of the patient when presented with new or different information

There are three types of preceptees who demonstrate poorly integrated knowledge.

1. **Type 1**—These preceptee are commonly described as being "in over their head." They attempt to solve problems or perform patient care tasks without adequate prerequisite learning experience (Hendricson & Kleffner, 2002). They are the victim of a nursing curriculum that emphasizes memorization of facts rather than using information to solve patient care problems, such as case

studies. They have spent many hours in class lectures but are not prepared to either assess or care for patients. They are unable to answer even the simplest of questions posed to them by a preceptor. These preceptees may also not have taken advantage of learning opportunities afforded to them but were promoted anyway.

2. **Type II**—These preceptees are progressing along the novice to expert learning continuum but are situated at the stage where their knowledge base is fragmented and still developing.

3. **Type III**—These preceptees may have difficulties beyond the normal issues of the novice to expert learner.

Preceptors and educators can help preceptees move from novice to expert by questioning them to build critical thinking. This is reviewed in the chapter on critical thinking skills. These questions from the preceptor allow the preceptee to think and gather bits of information learned through their previous clinical and didactic experiences. The preceptee is then able to verbalize to the instructor or preceptor their understanding of the information. Questioning such as that used to build critical thinking skills is termed "connecting the dots."

### Is the Preceptee Aware That They Have Limited Knowledge and Skills?

Some preceptees fall into a category aptly named "unskilled and unaware of it" (Hendricson & Kleffner, 2002). They reach false conclusions when discussing patient care, are unable to perform nursing tasks accurately, and are unaware of their incompetence. However, these preceptees are in denial and often are overconfident and arrogant. These individuals have poorly developed metacognition, meaning they lack the ability to distinguish correct from incorrect actions. They are unable to, like most individuals, self-correct and refine their behavior (self-monitor). The majority of preceptees are able to understand that they do not know something and therefore do not place themselves or their patients in danger. Those with poor metacognition do. Preceptors become frustrated with these preceptees, and with good reason. These preceptees:

- Were rarely provided feedback in the past that would have assisted them.
- Do not learn from the feedback that is provided because it is not precise and is provided infrequently.
- Do not learn from observation as to how to function.

There has been some evidence to support that these preceptees will learn from debriefing. If they demonstrated poor clinical judgment, their actions can be verbally compared to correct actions so that the preceptee develops corrective skills.

## Does the Preceptee Have an Undiagnosed Learning Disability?

Many students proceed with their college courses with undiagnosed learning disabilities that may only be recognized by a professor or preceptor. It is rare, but it does occur. The preceptee may never have been subject to the level of reading and comprehension that they experience in nursing school, or they may have been able to cope in high school but are now faced with intense college courses and their adaption skills to the known disability may no longer work. You will very rarely see these signs in the preceptee that has graduated nursing school because it was addressed prior to graduation, but you may encounter a nursing student who has a learning disability.

Signs of an undiagnosed learning disability include:

- Difficulty reading out loud
- Difficulty understanding what they are reading
- Difficulty completing written tests (may be reported by faculty)
- Failure to follow written instructions
- Difficulty understanding flow charts, diagrams, and picture instructions
- Difficulty writing, unable to express thoughts or ideas in written format

If these issues occur alone, it is not necessarily a learning disability. Seen in combination or with other signs of poor clinical or classroom performance, however, it very often is. If you as the preceptor suspect a learning problem, contact the faculty immediately and speak to them in person. Do not discuss a potential learning disability via text or email. Your only responsibility is to alert the faculty. The school will follow up with the preceptee.

## Does the Preceptee Have Difficulty Performing Tasks or With Motor Skills?

You may observe a preceptee (usually a student nurse) who is unable to draw up medication through a syringe or any other skill or task involving fine motor skills. This may merely be the result of a lack of practice. If it continues, even with practice, it may be the result of a learning disability that affects eye-hand coordination, fine motor skills, and the brain's interpretation of tactile stimuli. Ways in which the preceptor can assist the student are:

- Allow the preceptee time to see and analyze all the tools they will be using to complete a patient care task (allow them to manipulate supplies)—can be done in a simulation lab or allow them to use a teaching kit rather than waste sterile supplies.
- Allow the preceptee to observe the preceptor complete the skill. The preceptor should speak their way through the task so that they are explaining what they are doing and why.
- Allow the preceptee to ask questions.
- Repeat the practice procedure if requested by the preceptee.
- Allow the preceptee to practice the skill; preceptors should provide immediate feedback.
- Compare what they have completed to the ideal (if errors were committed).
- Allow the preceptee to verbalize why they feel errors were committed.
- Preceptors should be specific in their feedback about how the skill completion can be improved.
- Allow the preceptee ample time for practice.

### Does the Preceptee Know How to Study?

Many students have reached college without learning effective study habits. You may encounter a nursing student, usually a freshman, who cannot transfer the knowledge acquired in their course work to the clinical area. To correct bad study habits, you may suggest to them:

- Study in a quiet area, away from distractions. Don't attempt to study while watching TV or listening to music.
- Try to study at a desk, not while lying down.
- Have a study plan and stick to it, don't allow others to distract you or make you deviate from your study plans. Sacrifice a social life now for the returns of good grades and successful course completion.
- Use multiple learning styles.
- Use time in the nursing skills lab to "back up" what is learned from lectures and reading.

- Write notes in class and review them.
- Ask questions during class and of clinical faculty.
- Read ahead and review *prior* to class so that you have questions prepared and a familiarity with the material to be covered.

## Is the Preceptee Being Given a Quality Learning Experience?

### Fast Facts

The preceptor is not responsible for what occurs in the nursing classroom. They are responsible for what happens in the clinical area and the education received by them.

Ensure that the preceptee is receiving a quality clinical preceptorship:

- Make the preceptee aware of the learning objectives of the preceptorship. Ensure that as a preceptor, you are clear as to what the preceptee is to be learning while with you.
- Does the preceptee know the method by which they will be evaluated? Review skills with them that they are to learn.
- Can you ascertain that what is learned in course work is immediately being observed in the clinical area? In other words, is new information backed up by a learning opportunity in clinical? Ask the preceptee or clinical faculty what the preceptee is learning. Endeavor to find a patient or experience matching the needed objectives.
- Closely monitor the patient as needed; don't leave them on their own when they are first on the unit or with practicing new skills. Do not allow them to find patients to care for on their own. Provide guidance in patient selection.
- Provide feedback (see Chapter 8, The Value of Feedback).
- Allow preceptees time to observe you and other nurses so that they can model care.

### Is the Preceptee Distracted?

"Life gets in the way" and preceptees not only must deal with the rigors of school but also their family and work obligations outside of the clinical area. If the preceptee is unusually distracted, anxious, or distressed, the preceptor may ask if there is anything troubling the preceptee. Often, they do not want to share any troubling issue, but if it obvious something is distracting them from their clinical work, you should share that with them. Share your concerns with the faculty as well as they might also have insight.

## What Is the Preceptee's Level of Competence?

Preceptees are knowingly and sometimes unknowingly moving through these stages. All preceptees enter the clinical learning area as an unconscious incompetent; they don't know what they don't know. However, as they become consciously incompetent, they become very aware of what they don't know and may become distressed. They realize this career they've chosen is not so easy to learn and they may experience negative "self-talk." They may see other preceptees who are in their class doing well and wonder why they themselves are struggling. They may begin to try to hide their lack of knowledge and come across as either being obnoxious in the clinical area or acting like they don't care.

This behavior is unconsciously displayed because the preceptee is afraid they will be found out. Preceptors should recognize this for what it is and assist the student by being encouraging, allowing practice time, being non-judgmental, and providing positive feedback. With time, the preceptee will emerge from this panicked stage and move onto the next phases.

A method used by medical faculty to assist medical students in the conscious incompetent stage is PET, or **Prime, Partition, Praise, Empathy, Expectations, Teach, Help and Model**

P—**Prime**—Before a preceptee begins a patient care task or performs a skill, *prime* them by verbally reviewing what skill they will be performing. Let them know of any potential patient problems that may occur. Ask the preceptee how they will deal with any problems should they occur.

P—**Partition**—Start the preceptorship with less acute patients and then move on to more acutely ill as the preceptorship proceeds.

P—**Praise**—Provide plenty of positive feedback! Positive feedback is great when things go well, but remember to encourage the preceptee when they are discouraged or encounter a problem.

E—**Empathy**—Be sure to share stories of your time in preceptorship including errors and other cringe-worthy events. Explain how you used these events to make you a better nurse. Be sure to emphasize that mistakes are a part of learning and that learning is a continuum that never stops.

**E—Expectations**—Be sure to always be aware of what your preceptee can and cannot do at any stage of preceptorship. This way you will avoid unreasonable expectations that will increase their anxiety.

**T—Teach**—Be an active preceptor who coaches, mentors, rehearses, and provides helpful feedback.

**H—Help**—You are there to assist the preceptee, so focus on teaching them, not so much on constantly evaluating their performance. They are there to learn. Help them to identify what they do not know and what they require assistance with. Always be on the lookout for new learning opportunities for them.

**M—Model**—How do you know what you are doing is correct? Allow one your nursing peers (or better yet a nurse educator) review your demonstration of a nursing skill. Also tell the preceptee what you are doing as you perform a skill.

## References

Hendricson, W. D., & Kleffner, J. H. (2002). Assessing and helping challenging students: Part one, why do some students have difficulty learning? *Journal of Dental Education, 66*(1), 43–61.

# 5

# Critical Thinking Skills

*All nursing faculty and staff development educators agree that the skill of critical thinking is essential in providing safe and comprehensive patient care. Although all educators agree on this point, they are unable to agree as to what actually defines critical thinking. Because of this lack of consensus, teaching someone how to think critically can be difficult. It follows, then, that if there is no clear definition of critical thinking and no agreed-upon curriculum, the determination of how to evaluate the skill in the preceptee is also unclear. Even more challenging is how to integrate critical thinking into everyday nursing practice. With all this in mind, it is still essential that the preceptee be taught to think critically and that their ability to do so be evaluated. Critical thinking, problem-solving, and decision-making are crucial to the practice of the registered professional nurse.*

After reading this chapter, the reader will be able to:

1. Define critical thinking
2. List the habits of critical thinkers
3. List three methods that promote critical thinking
4. List 10 teaching methods that promote critical thinking
5. List the steps of the Five-Minute Preceptor

## CRITICAL THINKING IN ACTION

Why do we have "rapid response teams"? For those new to nursing, rapid response teams have always existed. The overhead page is a normal occurrence, but it shouldn't be. "Failures in planning and communication, and failure to recognize when a patient's condition is deteriorating, can lead to failure to rescue and become a key contributor to in-hospital mortality" (Institute for Healthcare Improvement, n.d.). Nursing shortages, poorly developed educational activities, and insufficient organizational safety practices contribute to delayed responsiveness to deteriorating patients by bedside nurses (Subbe & Welch, 2013). Delayed intervention results in patient demise and disability, as well as increased financial burden for the patient and the organization (Chan et al., 2008; Leach & Mayo, 2013). The bedside nurse needs to quickly recognize the patient whose condition is rapidly deteriorating. They need to use their clinical judgment and critical thinking skills to confidently handle the crises and improve the outcome of the patient. In a nutshell, rapid response teams exist because nurses have lost the ability to think critically!

## WHAT IS CRITICAL THINKING?

The term *critical thinking* has been discussed in relation to how a nursing student or new nurse is performing. "Are they thinking critically?" is an often-heard phrase in clinical nursing education. But what is critical thinking? Everyone from Socrates to Jean Piaget has a different interpretation and definition of critical thinking. However, generally speaking, scholars agree that critical thinking involves the following:

- It is an interpretation or analysis of an issue or problem, followed by evaluation or judgment.
- It requires that a person have knowledge about a particular subject.
- It is not a natural skill and it takes time and effort to learn.
- A person must be "willing to pursue 'truth' to wherever it may lie, persist through challenges, evaluate [his or her] own thinking fairly, and abandon faulty thinking for new and more valid ways of reasoning" (Nilson, 2014).
- It is learned by answering "challenging, open-ended questions that require genuine inquiry, analysis, or assessment" (Nilson, 2014).

To think critically, the preceptee should be able to recognize patient care problems, identify alternative nursing interventions to provide care, and anticipate the outcomes of the care provided. Interventions should be based on the most current best practices. When preceptors ask questions of preceptees, they assist them in analyzing patient problems and finding the best possible solutions.

**Fast Facts**

"…merely teaching facilitation of critical thinking is insufficient; utilization requires ongoing support, education and reinforcement" (Cotter & Dienemann, 2016).

## HABITS, CHARACTERISTICS, AND COGNITIVE SKILLS OF CRITICAL THINKERS

According to Rubenfeld and Scheffer (2015), critical thinkers have the following habits, characteristics, and cognitive skills:

- Confidence—in their reasoning abilities
- Contextual perspective—to consider the whole of the situation, rather than just parts
- Creativity—to be able to think "outside the box," able to discover or restructure ideas
- Flexibility—to adapt, modify, or change thoughts, ideas, and behaviors
- Inquisitiveness—to actively seek new knowledge and understanding by multiple means
- Intellectual integrity—to seek the truth through honest processes
- Intuition—a sense of knowing without use of reason
- Open-mindedness—being open to different views and sensitive to own biases
- Perseverance—determination
- Reflection—looking back on an action to better understand and self-evaluate

Those who think critically have the following cognitive skills: analyzing, applying standards, discriminating, information seeking, logical reasoning, predicting, and transforming knowledge.

## HOW TO PROMOTE CRITICAL THINKING

There are several ways to promote critical thinking in the preceptee and there are multiple ways to hinder critical thinking as well. Promote discussion using the real-life situations presented in the unit. Avoid lecturing the preceptee about what could or should happen. Avoid answering all of the questions of the preceptee all of the time. Allow them time to think through and find the answers themselves. Make sure you have the means necessary for them to find the answer.

### Questioning (The Number One Strategy)

Questions should not be posed in rapid-fire succession or used to make the preceptee feel that they are not knowledgeable. On the contrary, questions should be used to elicit information and help the preceptee pull together information. They should never be used to embarrass the preceptee. The underlying purpose of the questions should be clarified until the preceptee becomes used to this teaching style. For example, the preceptor might state, "I'm going to ask you a series of questions that will help you reason through your care of the patient."

**Fast Facts**

Ask "why" and use open-ended questions to elicit information; it will lead to more questions that go into greater depth.

The nursing process is the basis for the care that we provide, and every nursing action should be addressed within that process, including critical thinking. The following list of questions can be used to elicit responses based on the nursing process, many of which are adapted from Twibell, Ryan, and Hermiz (2005).

*Assessment*
- "Tell me about your patient."
- "After assessing your patient, what other information do you feel that you need?"

- "What do you think is contributing to this lab (or test) result?"
- "What do your findings represent?"

### Planning

- "Based on your assessment, what are the nursing diagnoses you've assigned to this patient?"
- "What are some options in the care of this patient?"
- "What are the next steps you are going to perform for this patient?"
- "What do you hope to achieve for your patient with these planned steps?"
- "If you take these steps, what will happen?"
- "What might happen if you *don't* take these steps?"
- "Are the goals you have established for the patient measurable?"
- "Are the goals you have established for the patient attainable?"
- "Is there any aspect of care you can delegate to another member of the healthcare team"?
- Establish a priority list for the care of this patient. "What should be done immediately?" "What should be done next?" and so on.
- "What do you feel is the worst thing that may occur with this patient? If that was to occur, what are your plans to address it?"

### Implementation

- "Why are you completing _____ in this way?"
- "What action should you take right now?"
- "What are your plans for meeting the goals you have established for the patient?"
- "Why is this medication (treatment, lab work, etc.) needed?"
- "What are the side effects of this medication (treatment, etc.) What are the risks involved with this care?"
- "How will this medication (treatment, intervention) affect *this* patient?"
- "What assessment findings do you need to check prior to performing this action (e.g., obtaining vital signs, lab results)?"
- Prior to a skill being performed, ask why it is being done, how should it be done, what could happen if it is performed incorrectly, what precautions should be taken.
- "What can the nurse do to assist the patient through a particular situation?"
- "How can you act as the patient advocate in this situation?"
- "What patient and/or family teaching should take place?"

*Evaluation*

- "How do you know the actions you have taken have been effective?"
- "What signs and symptoms would the patient be demonstrating if they were getting worse/better?"
- "Name some problems that you might anticipate."
- "Did the interventions you performed for the patient affect them positively or negatively?"
- "What evidence can you provide to demonstrate that your plan of care was effective?"
- "After evaluation, what changes would you make to the plan of care?"
- "What data are you reviewing that prompted you to change your plan of action?"
- "How would you reprioritize your care?"
- "What did you find interesting about this case?"
- "Did anything unusual occur?"
- "Is there a difference between what you learned regarding this patient's diagnosis and/or expected outcomes and what actually occurred?"
- "What do you feel is the most important thing that you have learned from taking care of this patient?"

**Fast Facts**

If the preceptee is unable to answer the questions, the preceptor should begin again with basic questions and build back up to more complex questions.

## REVIEW OF DOCUMENTS, WRITTEN WORK, AND POLICIES AND PROCEDURES

It is helpful to have the preceptee review the written care plan already established by the nursing staff. By reviewing the care plan together, the preceptor can question the preceptee about different aspects of the plan. Even more helpful for the preceptee is for them to develop a care plan for the patient and then have the preceptor review the document and question the preceptee using the nursing process-related questions presented earlier. A few suggestions follow:

- Give the preceptee their assignment and ask the preceptee to review the patient record.
- Ask the preceptee to formulate a plan of care for the patient using principles learned in the classroom or clinical setting.
- Ask the preceptee what they think should be done and to explain the rationale for the action.
- If you are reviewing a care plan that has been completed by another nurse, ask the preceptee to identify any alternate or additional ways they feel care could be completed.

## CONFERENCES

Discussing the care that the preceptee will provide or has also already performed is important for the development of critical thinking. Use the following positive comments and behaviors when speaking with the preceptee:

- "Tell me what you think."
- "That's a great idea! Let's share it with others and see what they think."
- "You've heard the issue; do you have a different idea of how to solve it?"
- "If we do it that way, what are some of the possible outcomes?"
- "How did you come to this conclusion?"
- "Let's explore some options."
- "What are the possible reasons for _____?"
- "What would you do if _____ happened?" (You can also provide specific examples of a patient care issue and ask how the preceptee would handle the situation.)
- If a patient develops a condition or issue, ask the preceptee to draw a conclusion as to what may be causing the symptoms that are occurring. Also ask what assessments should be completed on the patient.
- Listen quietly, be patient, be enthusiastic.
- Find out what motivates the preceptee and utilizes this in your teaching.
- Be confident in the preceptee's ability and skills.
- Acknowledge and reward the preceptee when they use critical thinking skills. Document positive performance.

- Have high standards and do not deviate from them.
- Foster teamwork on the unit and with other healthcare team members.
- If an error occurs, point out what was right and then work to improve the system that may have led to the error.
- Use real-life case studies and stories.
- Assist the preceptee in getting involved with their profession.
- Encourage the use of the SBAR system (see Chapter 7, Prioritization and Communication, and the form in Chapter 16, Preceptorship Competency Forms and Clinical Tools), which is an excellent format for critical thinking and planning of care.
- Help the preceptee discover new knowledge through research, questioning, and discovery.

### Still More Ways...

To think critically, nurses must be capable of three actions: thinking ahead, thinking in action, and thinking back (Nurse Preceptor Academy, 2008). Break these down by encouraging the following lines of action and inquiry:

- **Thinking Ahead:** The preceptee must be proactive and be able to plan ahead for any complication or patient issue that could occur. Encourage this ability by asking:
    - "What complications could occur in this patient?"
    - "What issues will you have to manage?"
    - "What supplies or resources will you need to care for the patient?"
- **Thinking in Action:** The preceptee must be able to think while caring for the patient or think on their feet in the midst of stress. Encourage this ability by having the preceptee plan a simple procedure through to its conclusion, including assessments, gathering of supplies, and postprocedure assessment. Review with the preceptee the reasons the procedure is needed, the steps of the procedure, any potential problems and risks, and finally, any solutions to any problems that may occur.
- **Thinking Back:** The preceptee also needs to be able to think back to the actions that were taken in caring for a patient. They need to be able to reason and analyze why these actions were taken and whether anything could have been done differently. Asking the following questions will help in this analysis:
    - "What was the most important patient issue to consider?"

- "Was the most important issue addressed?"
- "Of the facts that you have gathered, which was most important? Tell me why."

## Fast Facts

Another method of teaching critical thinking is to tell the preceptee what you are thinking and why you are doing what you are doing. Talk to them as you are performing a procedure, completing care, and so on. For example, you might state "I'm doing this because _____." "I anticipate that this will happen, so I'm doing _____."

## DOES YOUR TEACHING STYLE PROMOTE CRITICAL THINKING?

As a preceptor, your actions and teaching methods also influence how the preceptee learns critical thinking. Review your teaching style and ask the following of yourself:

- Do I evaluate the preceptee's thinking style and give credit for their thinking process (i.e., "thinking out of the box")?
- Am I confident in my reasoning ability?
- Am I inquisitive; do I look for answers and seek new knowledge?
- Do I use different techniques in teaching to appeal to different learning styles?
- Do I encourage multiple questions?
- Do I assist others in finding information and resources?
- Am I open-minded?
- Am I able to describe to the preceptee what I am thinking?
- Do I decrease the anxiety of the preceptee by explaining my actions and reviewing care prior to providing?
- Do I use humor in my teaching?
- Do I acknowledge that competency in performance goes beyond merely performing the skill (copying the skills of another) to include being able to transfer knowledge learned into action?
- Do I use mistakes as an opportunity to learn and grow?
- Do I ask the preceptee to expand their answers by using open-ended statements such as, "Tell me more…"?

- Do I encourage collaborative learning between myself and the preceptee, knowing that we can learn from each other?
- Do I allow and encourage the preceptee to teach me?

## THE FIVE-MINUTE PRECEPTOR

Medical schools have been utilizing a technique called the One-Minute Preceptor (OMP) to ascertain their students' current knowledge level, cognitive process, and perceived plan of care. The medical preceptor can then provide immediate feedback within a short period of time. This method is not appropriate for use during basic nursing education and preceptorship because medical and nursing care is not interchangeable. Nurses must plan their care of the patient, incorporating aspects for all professions involved with the patient. Bott, Mohide, and Lawlor (2011) changed the OMP principles, incorporating nursing processes and wording, and extended the time frame to better encompass all that the nurse must consider in the patient's plan of care. Thus, the Five-Minute Preceptor was developed. The tool should be used when a specific situation is occurring with a patient, not for general information about the patient. (See Chapter 16, Preceptorship Competency Forms and Clinical Tools, for further information.)

## ARE THEY THINKING CRITICALLY?

You can determine if your preceptee is thinking critically by asking questions and observing behaviors. Review your preceptorship evaluation tools. Are critical thinking indicators built into them? If not, recommend that they are updated. Use the Critical Thinking Evaluation Check-Off List in Chapter 16, Preceptorship Competency Forms and Clinical Tools, to assess the preceptee's critical thinking skills.

## HOW TO *NOT* PROMOTE CRITICAL THINKING IN THE PRECEPTEE

Unfortunately, there are many nurses who don't think creatively or innovatively, don't act on their assessment findings, don't follow up on a change in patient condition, or don't advocate for their patients.

These nurses may be using "traditional thinking" and have poor critical thinking skills. Elements of traditional thinking are found among the following list of ways to *not* promote critical thinking in your teaching style.

- Not learning from mistakes made by yourself or others
- Demanding that nothing changes; the "we've always done it this way" attitude
- Treating each patient issue in isolation rather than attempting to see how this action connects to other issues or causes
- Not connecting events with knowledge
- Not seeing beyond what is possible in the future
- Solving problems in isolation
- Demanding that things be done your way and no other
- Completing a task for the preceptee instead of allowing them to do so
- Allowing personal dislikes and prejudices to cloud your judgment
- Having a lack of self-confidence
- Having poor communication and documentation skills, and not working well with others
- Not furthering your personal education in both nursing and beyond
- Imposing strict time limitations on decision-making

What you say and the behaviors you model to preceptees stay with them long after the preceptorship and will affect them far into their nursing careers. We've all heard negative comments in our nursing education and perhaps used them ourselves on fellow staff or preceptees. Using the following statements when speaking to a preceptee (or any staff member) will stifle their thinking, learning, and creativity and negatively impact their self-esteem. Imagine the impact on patient care as well.

- "That's a dumb idea" or "That's a stupid question!"
- "We've always done it this way here" and "That won't work here."
- "You ask too many questions!"
- "It's too complicated, so I'll just show you."
- "Just memorize how to do this and don't deviate."
- "You spend too much time with your patients."
- "We've tried that and it didn't work."
- "I can't believe they didn't teach you that."

Also avoid nonverbal signs of boredom, anger, frustration, or irritation, such as eye-rolling, smirking, sighing, finger-tapping, or constantly looking at a watch or clock.

## EVIDENCE-BASED NURSING PRACTICE

Evidence-based practice (EBP) involves consciously using current best practice (clinical expertise, backed up by best available research evidence and taking into consideration patient and family preferences) in making well-informed decisions in the care of the patient. For years, schools of nursing and staff development have been teaching tradition-based nursing skills because "that's how it's always been done."

Now, nursing is systematically analyzing current skills and care practices in light of best research evidence and ensuring that they are scientifically-based. Schools of nursing and staff development are obligated to teach scientifically based skills and procedures, and this has changed the way we teach nursing in the clinical area. You must ensure what you are teaching is evidence based and not tradition based. In doubt about where to find the best possible literary sources of evidence-based nursing for your practice area? Follow the guidelines listed in Chapter 16, Preceptorship Competency Forms and Clinical Tools.

### Remember

- Although schools of nursing have revamped their curriculums to reflect these changes, there are still practicing nurses who are not aware that skills and procedures have been updated. Before allowing another nurse to oversee your preceptee, ensure that what they are teaching reflects EBP.
- EBP has been proven to improve patient outcomes.
- EBP decreases unnecessary procedures and treatments.
- EBP decreases complications from procedures and treatments.
- EBP expands a nurse's skill level.

### References

Bott, G., Mohide, E. A., & Lawlor, Y. (2011). A clinical teaching technique for nurse preceptors: The five minute preceptor. *Journal of Professional Nursing, 27*(1), 35–42. doi:10.1016/j.profnurs.2010.09.009

Chan, P. S., Khalid, A., Longmore, L. S., Berg, R. A., Kosiborod, M., & Spertus, J. A. (2008). Hospital-wide code rates and mortality before and after implementation of a rapid response team. *JAMA, 300*(21), 2506–2513. doi:10.1001/jama.2008.715

Cotter, E., & Dienemann, J. (2016). Professional development of preceptors improves nurse outcomes. *Journal for Nurses in Staff Development, 32*(4), 192–197. doi:10.1097/NND.0000000000000266

Institute for Healthcare Improvement. (n.d.). Rapid response teams. Retrieved from http://www.ihi.org/Topics/RapidResponseTeams/Pages/default.aspx

Leach, L. S., & Mayo, A. M. (2013). Rapid response teams: qualitative analysis of their effectiveness. Retrieved from https://www.semanticscholar .org/paper/Rapid-response-teams%3A-qualitative-analysis-of-their -Leach-Mayo/e4b06ae7ce1cbff86f816ac20fc0a594fd6f950d

Nilson, L. B. (2014, December 1). Unlocking the mystery of critical thinking. *Faculty Focus.* Retrieved from www.facultyfocus.com/articles/ instructional-design/unlocking-mystery-critical-thinking/

Nurse Preceptor Academy. (2008, April). Critical thinking from three perspectives; and critical thinking: What does it look like? *Preceptor News, 2.* Retrieved from https://www.nursingcenter.com/cearticle?an=00124645 -201207000-00014&Journal_ID=54029&Issue_ID=1400165

Rubenfeld, M. G., & Scheffer, B. K. (2015). *Critical thinking tactics for nurses: Achieving the IOM competencies* (3rd ed.). Boston, MA: Jones & Bartlett Learning.

Subbe, C. P., & Welch, J. R. (2013). Failure to rescue: Using rapid response systems to improve care of the deteriorating patient in hospital. *Journal of Patient Safety and Risk Management, 19*(1), 6–11. doi:10.1177/1356262213486451

Twibell, R., Ryan, M., & Hermiz, M. (2005). Faculty perceptions of critical thinking in student clinical experiences. *Journal of Nursing Education, 44*(2), 71–79. doi:10.3928/01484834-20050201-06

# 6

# Organizing the Clinical Day

*One of the most difficult things you, as a preceptor, will do is "slow down my day and explain what I do." It is important to review with the preceptee how you structure a "typical" day on the unit. Understand that organizing the shift can take some time to perfect because, as we know, each patient care situation will adjust the nurse's focus and lead to a change in priorities throughout the day.*

After reading this chapter, the reader will be able to:

1. List five activities to perform prior to the first clinical day with the preceptee
2. List five activities to perform on the first clinical day
3. List 10 items the preceptee should perform prior to obtaining report
4. List 10 items the preceptee should perform after obtaining report
5. List five items to utilize when creating a patient assignment for the preceptee

## BEFORE THE FIRST CLINICAL DAY

The preceptor relationship begins before the first clinical day. The groundwork for the future is laid during the preceptee's facility orientation process or when the student is introduced to you by the nursing faculty. Be sure to define your role and how long the preceptorship period will last. This is also the time when you should communicate YOUR expectations for the preceptor experience. Share your belief that the preceptorship experience requires active participation on the part of the preceptee. Convey that you will provide a safe, nonthreatening learning environment and the preceptee will not be made to perform any skill or action that they have not been taught. The following recommendations and tips should help the preceptee's first clinical day to go as smoothly as possible. Always remember what it was like to be the new nurse or new to an area of nursing.

- Meet with the preceptee and introduce yourself. Seeing a familiar face on the first day of clinical will decrease the preceptee's stress level. If you can, meet for lunch or coffee!
- Tell the preceptee a little about yourself and your professional history. You can speak about how and why you became a nurse, your experiences with being new, and your role on the unit where the preceptorship will take place.
- Ask the preceptee to share with you their healthcare background or previous career and experiences and what they hope to learn during preceptorship.
- Reinforce with the preceptee when to arrive on the unit and where you will meet with him or her.
- Provide your contact information and how you can be reached. Make sure you have the preceptee's contact information as well.
- Mention a list of supplies that the preceptee should bring, especially if working in a facility that does not provide items such as blood pressure cuffs, thermometers, or pulse oximeters.
- Mention textbooks or apps that the preceptee may refer to during preceptorship, such as a unit specialty text (e.g., medical–surgical, orthopedic, oncology, etc.), drug book, or skills book, should these references not be computer-based at your facility.
- Provide a brief tour of unit and identify the location of locker room, staff room, break room, and so forth, as well as where the preceptee may place personal belongings.
- Introduce the preceptee to fellow staff and their roles.
- Complete all necessary paperwork that your facility or the academic institution requires.
- Review facility and unit policy and procedures to refresh your memory about basic concepts in order to share them with the preceptee.

- Review documentation guidelines for your facility and unit.
- Review all schedules with the staffing coordinator, nurse educator, or faculty. If there are any questions or concerns, clarify them prior to the start of preceptorship. Be sure that your scheduled days off coordinate with those of the preceptee. Ensure that there is a preceptor available to the preceptee should you not be able to work on a scheduled day. If possible, introduce the preceptee to the alternate preceptor.
- Let them know the policy of calling out sick and who they should contact if calling the unit.
- Make fellow staff aware you are precepting and are interested in skills and tasks that can be shared with the preceptee. So as to not overwhelm the preceptee, introduce them to staff slowly over the period of preceptorship.
- Try to not leave the preceptee alone socially during the first days of their experience; include them on meal and other breaks. Make sure that the preceptee feels welcome and is being made to feel as part of the team.
- Make sure they know the dress code of the unit/facility.
- Ensure that the new nurse employee is provided facility name tag/ employee identification, as well as a parking pass (if applicable) and all computer codes necessary for the completion of their work and documentation.

## THE FIRST CLINICAL DAY

Some of the items listed below apply not only to the first day but also throughout preceptorship. Briefly review how your ideal day is structured, including typical unit scheduling of meals and break times or other events such as patient care activities (particularly in long-term care and subacute facilities).

Be aware and understand the preceptee will be anxious. Assure the preceptee they will not be left alone in a new situation and you are there to give assistance and guidance. Reassure the preceptee anxiety is normal, but you will do what you can to alleviate anxiety and build confidence. Recommendations and tips to help minimize stress and anxiety on the part of the preceptee:

- Be aware of the preceptee's strengths and perceived weaknesses. The staff development instructor or faculty should share with you the results of competency assessments or clinical issues prior to the beginning of preceptorship. If that does not occur, you may ask the preceptee about what they perceive are their strengths or weaknesses. As stated previously, inquire as to how they feel they learn best and also how they like to receive feedback.

- Question the preceptee about their past work and school clinical experiences, and then select new clinical experiences based on those needs. For example, many new nurses or students have never given an intramuscular injection or inserted a urinary catheter outside of the simulation lab. Elicit help from fellow staff in notifying you when new clinical experiences occur. However, the preceptor, not a fellow staff nurse, should observe the nurse or student in any new skill.

- Use subjective statements of strengths and weaknesses and competency assessment as a starting point for planned observation of the preceptee during care. For example, the preceptee may state that they inserted a urinary catheter during a school clinical experience. Review the procedure with the preceptee and then allow them to perform it with minimal input from the preceptor. If the preceptee is successful and no break in technique has occurred, then no further involvement is required of the preceptor. However, if the preceptee breaks sterile technique during the procedure, or has any other issue, immediately stop the procedure. If time allows, review the procedure both in simulation and through review of the literature. Obtain further clinical experiences based on this objective finding.

- Discuss the preceptorship process, including how you plan to work together. For example:
  - If a patient emergency occurs, the preceptor will take over the care of the patient with the preceptee mainly observing.
  - The preceptee may perform skills in which competency has been assessed, but guidance will come from the preceptor.
  - Debriefings will take place, especially after a patient care incident. These will assist the preceptee in verbalizing questions regarding their observation and future role.
  - When caring for a preoperative patient, the preceptor may provide preop mediations but allow the preceptee to perform patient teaching first (after having reviewed material with the preceptor). With a future preoperative patient, the roles could reverse based on subjective or objective findings obtained by the preceptor.

- Review the preceptorship schedule and explain when you will be providing care, when you will be supervising care, and when you will step back and allow the preceptee to care for the patient assignment. The preceptee should not feel you are "hovering" but that you are there in case you are needed. The goal is for the preceptee to act in the role independently. Once the preceptee's competency has been tested, and you have observed the preceptee perform a skill for the first time or as needed and deemed them competent, you may then allow the preceptee to perform that task independently.

- Reinforce that you expect and welcome questions!
- Reinforce that you expect the preceptee to ask for assistance if they encounter a situation that is completely unfamiliar. *However,* explain that you also anticipate that the preceptee will investigate provided resources on their own (e.g., textbooks, apps, policy and procedure manuals, staff education on computer terminals, etc.) and will verify the information found with you.
- Be sure that the preceptee, if applicable, has all computer emergency medical records (EMR) and other access codes that are appropriate.
- Familiarize the preceptee with the location of patient safety equipment, including the automated external defibrillator (AED) and crash cart, emergency preparedness and disaster manuals, fire exits, and fire extinguishers, and make sure they understand the nurse's role in a fire or emergency on the unit, the location of safety data sheets (SDS), guidelines for using any chemicals in the work area, and how to properly report an incident, including facility online reporting. Review all emergency codes (fire, disaster, elopement, cardiac arrest, medical emergency, rapid response, in-house security issues, bomb threat, etc.). Explain their role in each situation.
- The goal is for the preceptee to fully participate in active learning experiences. Understand that the preceptee will be nervous and will wish to only observe in certain situations. An exception to this rule includes patient care emergencies.
- Allow the preceptee to work with all equipment that they will be using for patient care including IV and feeding pumps, glucometers, IV equipment, dressing supplies, and any other equipment and patient monitors special to the unit they may not have encountered during school or other training.
- Show the preceptee a patient clinical record or EMR. Explain how patient care information is organized, and allow the preceptee to review it and practice sample documentation. It is appropriate for the preceptee to review the medical record and for you to

question the preceptee as to their findings. This can be done before receiving report on a particular patient or if a patient care issue occurs.

■ Review all unit specific policies and procedures (including any unwritten protocols). Be sure the preceptee is clear on what patient care is expected on the unit.

**Fast Facts**

Strictly observational experiences should be kept to a minimum.

## THROUGHOUT PRECEPTORSHIP: RECOMMENDATIONS FOR EFFECTIVE ONGOING PRECEPTING PRACTICES

Below is a guide to review with the preceptee on how to organize the beginning of a shift. Adjust it to so it is applicable to a specific patient care area or specialty. If possible, retain the same patient assignment during preceptorship. This will allow the preceptee to utilize the nursing process, evaluate their care, and adjust plans of care as needed. This list has also been provided as a check-off list in Chapter 16, Preceptorship Competency Forms and Clinical Tools.

Explain to the preceptee how it is helpful to develop their own organizational "style." Some nurses use a notebook or clipboard; some facilities have personal digital assistants (PDAs). Encourage the preceptee to avoid documenting on multiple pieces of paper, paper towels, sheets, and alcohol wipe labels. Although handy in an emergency, these dashed-off notes can get lost, setting the preceptee back even further in their schedule. Whatever the style, the preceptee should not rely on memory and instead should write down the care that has been planned and performed.

### Prior to Obtaining the Report

■ Check orders written in the past 24 hours and any orders or treatments that need to be carried out during the shift.
■ Check schedules for therapy and surgery. Explain the need to know if any preoperative or pretherapy medications are scheduled. (Do any patients require pain medication before therapy? Are there treatments that must be completed before the patient leaves the unit?)

- Check the patient's armband and ask the patient to identify themselves.
- Introduce yourself to the patient. If there is a whiteboard present in the patient's room, write your name and all other pertinent information as per unit policy.
- Briefly assess the patient's orientation, general condition, stability, and environment. Ensure that there are no immediate problems and note anything to address in report.
- Ascertain any immediate patient needs such as request for pain medication.
- Write down the needs or questions of the patient to refer to during and after report.
- Check the medication administration record for the medications scheduled to be administered during the shift. (When were as-needed [PRN] medications last administered? Are you knowledgeable regarding the medication?)
- Make sure that all medications that are to be administered during your shift are present. Verify if any are missing. Notify the pharmacy or follow unit procedure for obtaining the medication.
- Note if there are dressing changes or other wound care that must be completed during the shift, and how often.
- Note what other treatments must be completed during the shift. Explain to the preceptee what treatments and activities are completed by the nursing staff and which ones are completed by other members of the health care team.

## At the Bedside Following Report

- Make lists of what must be completed during the shift. Include dressing changes and other treatments and the number of times they must be completed during the shift.
- Complete either a focused or more thorough head-to-toe assessment. Begin with patients who may be leaving the unit for a test, therapy, or surgery, or the newly admitted patient.
- If a problem or issue is noted, address it immediately before continuing. Impart that small problems tend to snowball into larger ones unless handled immediately if possible.
- Reinforce to the preceptee that when they are speaking to the patient, mental status, skin color, breathing effort, and facial symmetry should also be assessed.
- The patient assessment should include anything "attached" to the patient, including intravenous lines, enteral feedings, urinary catheters, chest tubes, suction, drains, wound vacs, and so on.

- Ensure all monitors, pumps, specialty beds, and other patient care equipment is working correctly. If a malfunction is noted, the situation should be investigated and corrected. Review the procedure for removing medical equipment from service.

- Ensure the current intravenous solution is correct and infusing at the proper rate. What is the LIB ("left in bottle/bag")? Is a sufficient amount left for assessment rounds to be completed before hanging the next bag? Is the next bag ready to be hung? Confirm the pump is plugged in or charged. Follow facility policy, if applicable, for zeroing out the total infused on intravenous and enteral feedings so that it begins at "0" for the shift.

- Trace lines and tubing back to the patient and assess insertion sites, noting any signs of inflammation and infection.

- Note the amount of suction, urinary drainage, wound drainage, and so on. Noting the amount, consistency, odor, and color of any drainage is an important part of assessment and provides a baseline for future assessment.

- Perform a safety check. Place the call light within reach, and place the bed in the lowest position. Follow facility guidelines for use of side rails.

- Place necessary or frequently used belongings or necessary items within easy reach of the patient (e.g., glasses, tissues, phone, and water).

- Ensure the floor is not cluttered and any wires do not pose a tripping hazard.

- Look at the big picture. Abnormal findings need to be taken into consideration along with the rest of the assessment findings and results. Look for patterns.

- Compare the body for asymmetry/symmetry (e.g., the chest while breathing or the face when smiling).

- Compare one side of the body to the other (e.g., one leg to the other if edematous, one hand to the other if swollen, and one pulse site to the other if the other is weak or absent).

- Make notations regarding patient requests, including PRN medications. Inform the patient if they are not due for medication and when it will be available. Follow up on any patient requests.

### After Checking All Patients

The preceptee should:

- Document initial patient findings.
- Communicate abnormal findings appropriately.

- Prioritize activities for the shift (see Chapter 7, Prioritization and Communication).
  - Determine who is in immediate need of any PRN-type medications or treatments, then write this down and follow up immediately!
  - Complete and follow up on all urgent patient care issues.
  - Complete, earlier in the shift, other tasks and activities that they find uncomfortable or may not like performing. Putting off these issues will cause stress during the shift and make the preceptee feel that they have fallen behind.
  - Be sure not to procrastinate! It causes stress and delays tasks that must be accomplished.
  - Note tasks that can be quickly accomplished and those that may take longer.
  - Note tasks that must be completed at exact specified times, such as insulin administration.
- Follow up on all delegated tasks. Request feedback from the team member and follow up on any issues (see Chapter 8, The Value of Feedback).
- Ask for help if they get bogged down in patient care, and delegate the tasks and activities that can be handed off to others.
- After care is provided, prioritize again. What remains to be completed?
- Document as they go. Finding the time throughout the shift to document will save time at the end of the shift.

## Fast Facts

Remind the preceptee to follow the same system every day; otherwise they may potentially miss an important finding.

## CREATING A PATIENT ASSIGNMENT

Usually the emphasis for the student nurse while in school was on developing a plan of care based on information provided (e.g., medical diagnosis, brief history, and medication list) by their instructor. Researching the patient chart may not have been done before initiating the care of the patient; thus, the student was unable to review all aspects of care from different specialties. The student may not have been able to tie the past medical history to the patient's current medical condition. Perhaps the student did not see the value of the practices of other professions and the care they provided documented in their notes. Couple this with the fact many nursing students have had only a few hours one clinical day per week in which to carry out their interventions. There was no chance for follow up, evaluation, or reassessment. If this was the case with the preceptee, begin to develop in them the sense that nursing care should be based on a broader view or understanding than that of just the medical diagnoses. Preceptorship is a chance for the preceptee to develop clinical reasoning abilities. Give the preceptee the tools necessary to do so.

In creating a patient assignment, guide the preceptee to perform the following actions:

- Have the preceptee research a patient chart or EMR and develop a care plan.
- Have them list nursing diagnoses and the nursing interventions for each. Be sure that goals are measurable.
- Have the preceptee prioritize (see Chapter 7, Prioritization and Communication the patient's nursing diagnoses and verbalize the rationale for how they established priority.)
- Have the preceptee enact the care plan and evaluate the effectiveness of their interventions.
- Allow the preceptee the opportunity to interact with fellow health care providers in carrying out the plan.
- Have the preceptee evaluate the effectiveness of the plan and reassess and reprioritize.
- Ask the preceptee: "What are the goals you are attempting to attain (e.g., new skill, review of current skills, and so on)?" Create an assignment based on these goals.
- Begin with the patient assignment number the preceptee had in school before they graduated. Unfortunately, you may find this was one or two patients, or that the preceptee performed as a "team nurse" and never acted as a primary nurse for a group of patients. The preceptee also may have never delegated care to aides or other health care workers (see chapter on delegation); therefore, this skill will also have to be developed.
- Only assign less complicated patients at the beginning of preceptorship, leaving the patients with more complex care needs for later on in the process.

- Introduce the preceptee to the patients, assuring the patient that if the preceptee is a student, the preceptor is available at all times and that the preceptor is still guiding their care.
- When the preceptee has gained confidence with the current level of patients, increase the patient assignment by one to two patients. Carefully observe the preceptee as they care for the increased number. You may need to adjust the number of patients back by one or two patients until the preceptee gains confidence, and then adjust upward again.
- Allow the preceptee to care for the increased number of patients for several shifts until confidence has been reached and then increase the assignment number again.
- The ultimate goal is for the preceptee to confidently and safely care for the number of a given patient assignment similar to that of a typical staff nurse on your unit and sustain this number until the end of preceptorship. The preceptor should move from a position of assisting with care to observing the care the preceptee provides.
- Communicate with fellow staff or receive report from unit manager or charge nurse regarding the unit population. If you are focusing on a new skill to be learned or review of a current skill, then work this new skill into the day's schedule.
- Accompany the preceptee during all skills that are being performed for the first time. For example, the first time the preceptee passes medications or changes a dressing, they should be accompanied by the preceptor.
- Be aware of classes or skill/competency development being offered by staff development. Allow time for the preceptee to attend these classes.
- Allow time at the end of the day for review or debriefing of the day—what was learned, what needs to be reviewed, and problems or issues that arose. Debriefing the preceptee is critical to immediately address issues and promote critical thinking.
- Do not leave the preceptee on the unit alone at the end of the shift. If the preceptee is still completing work on the assignment, assist them.

# II

# Components of
Effective Preceptorship

# 7

# Prioritization and Communication

*Nursing care is complex, and teaching the preceptee how to correctly organize, prioritize, and make decisions is essential to the safety and quality of care that patients receive. Prioritization is simply the ability to differentiate between patient issues that require immediate attention and those issues that can wait. If a nurse is unable to differentiate between the two, then patient safety is at risk.*

After reading this chapter, the reader will be able to:

1. Explain the SBAR communication system
2. List five activities that will assist the preceptee with phone skills
3. Define the term cognitive stacking
4. List the CURE hierarchy
5. List four questions the preceptor can ask the preceptee that will assist with prioritization

## COMMUNICATION AMONG HEALTHCARE PROFESSIONALS

Many instances of poor communication result in patient injury and death. Older studies found that up to 80% of medical errors were related to communication issues, and others have shown half of communication breakdowns occur during patient "handoffs." Handoffs occur when one healthcare professional reports to another at either change of shift or transition of care (transfer from unit to unit or facility to facility), when there is a change of shift from nurse to nurse, or when there is communication between physicians.

One method used to reduce the incidence of missed communication is the SBAR technique. Developed by the U.S. Navy, the SBAR method was adopted by the healthcare industry in the 1990s. SBAR is an acronym that stands for situation, background, assessment, and recommendation, and it helps to structure the information being communicated to healthcare professionals about changes in a patient's condition:

- **S—Situation**: What is happening at the present time? Should be briefly and concisely stated
  - The nurse should begin by identifying themselves and the location.
  - The nurse should state the patient's name and the problem about which the nurse is calling.
  - The nurse should verbalize what has been assessed and what changes in the patient's status have been discovered.
- **B—Background**: What were the circumstances leading up to this situation? Brief and related to the current situation.
  - The nurse should give a brief history and current symptoms.
  - The nurse should include neurological, cardiovascular, respiratory, gastrointestinal, and genitourinary status; current lab work (compare to past lab work if relevant; e.g., current hemoglobin/hematocrit levels to previous or current drug levels to previous); current medications; and intravenous lines, if pertinent.
- **A—Assessment**: What is your basic assessment of the patient? What have you found? What do you think?
  - The nurse should state what the problem may or may not be.
  - The nurse should state whether the patient is deteriorating.
  - If the patient is unstable, the nurse should state what action must be taken.
- **R—Recommendation**: What are your recommendations to the MD or other healthcare professionals? State what you want for the care of the patient.

- The nurse should ask, "What should we do to correct the problem? I request that you … (transfer to critical care; come see the patient; order lab work, other tests, medications)."
- If the patient does not get better, the nurse should consider when to recontact the MD.
- Remind the nurse to read back recommendations and new orders.

## Fast Facts

Many new nurses and students consider SBAR to be an organizational tool. It assists them in charting and focusing on what is important in the care of patients, and in communicating patient needs to the physician and other healthcare personnel.

The Institute for Healthcare Improvement has an excellent website containing SBAR resources, toolkits, and forms. Locate them here: http://www.ihi.org/resources/Pages/Tools/SBARToolkit.aspx. A competency form is also located in Chapter 16, Preceptorship Competency Forms and Clinical Tools.

## PHONE SKILLS

After the nurse has gathered the assessment information on the patient, if necessity warrants, the information must be communicated to the appropriate healthcare provider. (Never mind about a patient crashing or coding; often one of the most stressful and daunting tasks to a preceptee is speaking on the phone with a physician!)

### Deciding to Call

- Assure the preceptee that knowing when or under what circumstances to call an MD comes with experience. If the preceptee is unsure whether a call should be made, remind them to first ask the preceptor, charge nurse, unit manager, or a nurse with whom they have a relationship on the unit.

■ Note that an RN may be asked to call an MD for another nurse. Remind the preceptee that they should always thoroughly investigate a situation before calling the MD to be sure that all the information that must be conveyed is on hand.

■ It may be best for the nurse to receive a mini "report" from the colleague who is asking for the call to be made so that the calling nurse is familiar with the case.

### Preparing for the Call

■ Practice with the preceptee what they are going to say on the phone prior to making a call.

■ Have the preceptee write down what they want to say or use a blank SBAR form.

■ Use instances in which other nurses assess their patients and decide to contact an MD as teaching moments for your preceptee. What would the preceptee do or say in the same instance?

■ Have your preceptee listen on the phone while you call an MD. Be sure the preceptee notes the information you are sharing and how you are interacting with the MD.

■ The preceptee should have all the information they need prior to calling an MD. They should try not to place an MD or any other healthcare professional on hold while scrambling to obtain necessary information.

### Calling the MD

■ The preceptor can listen on the phone while the preceptee speaks on the phone to an MD or other healthcare worker. The preceptor can fill in information missed by the preceptee by prompting them. The preceptor can also critique the telephone skills of the preceptee.

■ Remind the preceptee to always identify themselves and the facility when making a call to any MD, healthcare facility, testing facility, and so on.

■ Remind the preceptee that the individual to whom they are speaking may not be familiar with the patient (e.g., a covering MD); thus, the caller should always ask, "Do you know this patient?" or "Are you familiar with this patient?"

- The call to an MD or other healthcare professional should be documented as follows:
  - The time and with whom the preceptee spoke should be noted. Orders received should be noted (or the fact that no orders were received).
  - If multiple phone calls are made or messages left with a service or office, but the MD has not been reached, this must be documented as well.
  - If the preceptee is unable to contact an MD and has called multiple times or left multiple messages, review the policy regarding who should be notified and the chain of command.

### Issues in Calling the MD

- At some point in their professional careers, preceptees may encounter a rude MD or other healthcare professional while speaking on the phone. The preceptee should not retaliate by being rude, too. Advise the preceptee to:
  - Be calm and polite.
  - State what they need to say in order to obtain a necessary order for the patient or to provide needed information.
  - Report the incident to the nurse manager or supervisor.
- Role play with the preceptee in order to simulate a conversation that may include conflict with an MD or other health professionals. Scenarios could include advocating for the patient or sharing vital results needed for immediate orders.

### Fast Facts

Remind the preceptee that they are the patient advocate and information must be shared in order to provide quality care for the patient.

## HOW "THINGS" GET MISSED

Researchers have found that several factors disrupt the work patterns of a nurse, including missing equipment and supplies, interruptions, waiting for needed resources, communication inconsistencies, and lack of time (Ebright, Patterson, Chalko, & Render, 2003). Nurses are constantly ordering and reordering care (prioritization) based on many factors, all while being interrupted by a variety of sources. The nurse's thought processes, including the prioritization of care and the ability to carry out that care, are disrupted. In addition, outside factors such as missing equipment, supplies, medication that must be searched for and obtained, short staffing, and other everyday factors create additional obstacles to care and increase the risk to patient safety.

Beatrice Kalisch, in her 2006 report *Missed Nursing Care: A Qualitative Report*, noted different patient care activities that were often "missed" by nurses. This study was updated in 2017 to include results of hospital and staff surveys. Registered nurse reporting of patient care that is "missed" includes:

- Medications administered on time
- Ambulation as ordered
- Mouth care
- Turning and positioning
- Delayed or missed feedings or feeding patient when the food is still warm
- Patient education
- Response to call light within 5 minutes
- Emotional support to patient and/or family
- Hygiene (patient bathing/skin care)

The RNs in Kalisch's 2006 report gave the following reasons for the missed care: staffing issues, the time required for a particular nursing intervention, poor use of existing resources, and ineffective delegation. The reasons given then are the same today, but now include fatigue, burnout, multitasking, interruptions, compassion fatigue, complacency, and communication issues (Kalisch, 2017). Kalisch found what we all know to be true: "When nurses cannot or do not provide acceptable care, they are more dissatisfied with their jobs than would be true for employees who do not have these values and service orientation" (2017).

Patients recognize when their care is missed. When surveyed, patients noted when they did not receive mouth care or ambulation, when they were not assisted out of bed to a chair, when they were not bathed or provided information on tests/procedures. This is care they were aware of, and as you are reading this you are probably unconsciously listing nursing care you know was missed but that the patient was unaware. Missed nursing care not only affects the job satisfaction of the nursing staff, but more importantly, patient safety. Missed care can lead to anything from onset of delirium, pressure ulcers, falls, pneumonia, increased pain, thrombosis, urinary tract infections, muscle wasting, and death.

Krichbaum et al. (2007) investigated an experience they called "complexity compression." This occurs when RNs are expected to take on additional unplanned tasks and activities in a shorter time frame while also completing their planned work.

Nurses not only use their clinical, medical, scientific, pharmacological, and nursing process knowledge to make decisions regarding the care that they deliver, they also use their knowledge about the unit on which they work, availability of resources (staff and equipment), coworker relationships, and system processes. This knowledge, together with the current status of their patient, is used to make decisions regarding what and how to deliver nursing care.

According to Ebright et al. (2003), nurses have developed strategies to deal with factors that make their work difficult. These strategies include the following, and they should be encouraged by the preceptor:

- Thinking ahead
- Behaving proactively
- Employing strategic delegation
- Using handwritten or computerized notes for remembering and tracking care ("to-do lists")
- "Stacking" (also known as cognitive stacking)

Added to this are:

- Routinization
- Use of CURE hierarchy

## STRATEGIES DEFINED

Cognitive stacking is an invisible and dynamic process in which nurses organize and reorganize their activities according to changes and priorities throughout their shift. (Kohtz, Gowda, & Guede, 2017).

It allows the nurse to prioritize care that requires immediate attention and to form a mental list of remaining patient care needs (Kohtz et al., 2017).

Cognitive stacking is used to:

- Anticipate care to be given during the shift (even before arriving for the shift)
- Determine what care is possible given the resources and equipment available
- Determine when and how the care is to be delivered

Nurses perform this cognitive work constantly during the clinical day. How successfully this is accomplished (or not) will influence everything from work environment, quality of care, and safe patient outcomes to recruitment and retention of new nursing staff. It is necessary to understand how nurses perform this cognitive work in order to instill these skills in the preceptee.

Experienced nurses will arrive on the unit already forming a mental list of care and activities that will take place as they begin their shift. (Many of these items are found on the list in Chapter 6, Organizing the Clinical Day, and the competency list in Chapter 16, Preceptorship Competency Forms and Clinical Tools.) This mental list together with immediate observations, such as their patient assignment (including number of patients, their diagnosis, and location on the unit) and other unit related duties (e.g., narcotic count, supply inventory, crash cart check, etc.), are the basis of the prioritization list. Each patient assessment, observation, patient request, MD request/order, health care team member request, and care encounter adds to the continuous reordering of initial priorities.

According to Ebright et al. (2003), many factors that the nurse encounters throughout the shift will influence their ability to "stack." These include:

- **An unpredictable world:** Traditional healthcare has been dominated by a predictable worldview, one that assumes that units, healthcare systems, and patient responses are relatively predictable. It also assumes that even when the outcome of a situation goes wrong, it is the fault of the healthcare worker. While this may be the case, the many potential causative factors may not be investigated and the "cure" for the problem is usually deemed to be reeducation of the nurse. Prompted by the publication of the The National Academies report, *To Err Is Human* (IOM, 1999), systems rather than individuals are being reviewed in order to increase the quality and safety of patient care.

- **Complexity science:** A complex adaptive system (CAS) is a system that can adapt to a changing environment. Ebright (2010) notes that complexity science can be used to explain the intricacy of nursing care delivery to one patient within the larger context of an assignment within a unit within a department and within a hospital. The system, the patient, and the nurse are "dynamic, interconnected, interdependent, adaptive, and diverse" (Ebright, 2010). CASs adapt and change when confronted with situations. Viewing nursing care through the lens of complexity science gives insight to the many challenges of nursing care. For example, if a nurse commits an error, an understanding of complexity science would help those reviewing the situation to focus on the broader details of what led to the error by assuming that multiple issues may have been contributing factors, rather than focusing on isolated actions of an individual.
- **Trade-offs:** Nurses manage continuous care of patients and unit-related activities. Nurses are rarely able to complete a task without interruption. "RNs provide nursing care in the midst of the continual trade-off decisions they make regarding the most important activity for the moment, how it should be done, and what can wait until later or not be done at all" (Ebright, 2010).
- **Mindfulness:** A nurse's ability to make safe, well-informed clinical decisions is based on the nurse's ability to pay attention to and respond to changing patient information. Many nurses, of course, do this successfully and deliver high-quality, safe care. The fact that patient care items are "missed" is often the result of trade-off decisions made by the nurse throughout the course of a shift (although how much so is not clear).

## Fast Facts

When decisions are "traded off," the results can place the safety of the patient at risk.

## ROUTINIZATION

Routinization "is the development of previously successful habits that have become a repeated and integrated approach to routine situations" (Kohtz et al., 2017). Nurses usually develop the habit of making lists and this is an integral part of routinization. Encourage your preceptee to utilize lists.

Routine situations:

- The unit layout or location of patient care and other rooms
- The patient names within their assignment
- Performing and receiving patient reports
- Reviewing the patient record
- Performing assessments
- Administering medications
- Documentation
- End-of-shift or unit-to-unit reporting.

Some facilities have pre-printed or computer-generated lists for the care of the patient; what is expected to take place during the shift and these may be personalized for each patient. The list should be revised as new situations arise. Share how you developed and organized your patient care lists. These lists can also be used during preceptorship periods to review care completed or not completed and what requires review.

## PRIORITIZATION

Prioritization is another skill primarily learned through time and clinical experience, and it is a part of critical thinking. First priority goes to what nursing action is deemed most important first, then next most important, and so on. All nurses learn Maslow's Hierarchy of Needs, addressing physiological needs of the patient (hunger, thirst, etc.) upward toward safety, security, and so on. Although this is logical, students and new nurses can become easily stressed and overwhelmed by the constant need to prioritize and reprioritize their care. They will go from caring for one or two patients to an entire assignment at the end of preceptorship. How can the preceptor prompt the new nurse to prioritize care without *telling* them what the priority should be? After reviewing a patient care situation with the preceptee, Nelson, in her 2010 article "Helping New Nurses Set Priorities," recommends utilizing the following questions to encourage critical thinking:

- "What are you going to do first? Why?"
- "Of all that you have to do, which task/activity is more important? Why?"
- "What could happen if you don't do this now?"
- "What is most important to the patient?"

### Fast Facts

The preceptor should return to this list of questions throughout the shift and when the preceptee is confronted with changing situations and patient care needs. These questions encourage the preceptee to make informed decisions regarding prioritizing care.

It should be emphasized that:

- The task that has the highest priority is completed first and that each task should be finished before another is begun.
- Remaining tasks and any new tasks should be reprioritized based on patient information and assessments completed.
- The preceptor should be available to assist the preceptee in redirecting and refocusing their thought processes throughout the shift.

A postconference review or "debriefing" after a patient care situation will also help to focus the preceptee on care that was administered and why. (For example, did the patient experience an emergency or a decline?) Prioritization can still be learned *after* the care was given by using these modified questions suggested by Nelson:

- "Tell me why you are doing (why you did) this."
- "Why did (didn't) you decide to intervene at this time?"
- "Why did you make this choice?"
- "What would happen if you'd missed this clue?"
  Review with the preceptee the Initial Organization Review Checkoff List located in Chapter 16, Preceptorship Competency Forms and Clinical Tools.

## A PRIORITY LIST: WHAT TO DO FIRST?

Always build in time at the beginning of a shift to create a prioritization list. One exercise to assist the preceptee in prioritization is for the preceptee to assign nursing diagnoses to their patients and, from that initial list, prioritize the care. Assist the preceptee in listing tasks in order of importance, as described in Table 7.1.

## ANOTHER WAY TO LOOK AT IT

Another way to teach prioritization is to utilize the CURE hierarchy or the normative hierarchy The CURE hierarchy is as follows:

**C for Critical patient needs**—These are situations that require immediate nursing intervention to prevent significant patient deterioration and or death. This includes respiratory distress, chest pain, and changes in level of consciousness (Kohtz et al., 2017).

**U is for Urgent patient needs**—These are conditions that if not addressed may be harmful or cause significant discomfort. This includes not answering a fall alarm, administering as needed pain medications, clarifying healthcare provider orders (Kohtz et al., 2017).

**R is for Routine patient needs**—These include routine patient assessments and administering medications.

Table 7.1

| Priority Listing | |
|---|---|
| **High-priority tasks** | Tasks that, if not done immediately, will both threaten patients' safety or survival and require immediate nursing intervention. |
| **Second-level tasks** | Usually cases of untreated medical problems that require immediate attention, such as reporting abnormal lab work, treating acute pain, or threats to patient safety. |
| **Third-level tasks** | Everyday nursing activities and tasks, including such things such as monitoring medication side effects, patient teaching, and assisting with activities of daily living. |

**E is for Extras**—These are patient care activities that are not essential but that do promote patient comfort.

Normative hierarchy resembles the CURE hierarchy but provides further breakdown of tasks, including those activities to relieve pain and to complete normal nursing responsibilities such as dressing changes, administering medications, discharge planning, patient admission, documentation, assisting co-workers, patient teaching, stocking supplies, and personal times.

## Fast Facts

Consider your patient assignment; typically, the closer a patient is to their day of admission or postoperative day, the higher their acuity and risk for change in status. If there are no other critical patient issues with your assignment, then recent admitted and recent surgical patients should be assessed first. Patients with multi-body system disease involvement are complex. Again, if there are no other critical patient issues with your assignment, assess this type of patient first.

## References

Ebright, P. (2010). The complex work of RNs: Implications for healthy work environments. *Online Journal of Issues in Nursing.* Retrieved from www.nursingworld.org/MainMenuCategories/ANAMarketplace/ANA Periodicals/OJIN/TableofContents/Vol152010/No1Jan2010/Complex -Work-of-RNs.html

Ebright, P., Patterson, E., Chalko, B., & Render, M. L. (2003). Understanding the complexity of registered nurse work in acute care settings. *Journal of Nursing Administration, 33*(12):630–638. doi:10.1097/00005110-200312000 -00004

Institute of Medicine. (1999). *To err is human: Building a safer healthcare system.* Washington, DC: National Academies Press.

Kalisch, B. J. (2006). Missed nursing care: A qualitative study. *Journal of Nursing Care Quality, 21,* 306–313. doi:10.1097/00001786-200610000-00006

Kalisch, B. J. (2017, January). *Errors of omission: Missed nursing care.* NCSBN Annual Institute of Regulatory Excellence Conference, Clearwater Beach, FL.

Kohtz, C., Gowda, C., & Guede, P. (2017). Cognitive stacking: Strategies for the busy RN. *Nursing, 47*(1), 18–20. doi:10.1097/01.NURSE.0000510758 .31326.92

Krichbaum, K., Diemert, C., Jacox, L., Jones, A., Koenig, P., Mueller, C., & Disch, J. (2007). Complexity compression: Nurses under fire. *Nursing Forum, 42*(2), 86–94. doi:10.1111/j.1744-6198.2007.00071.x

Nelson, J. L. (2010). Helping new nurses set priorities. *American Nurse Today, 5*(5). Retrieved from www.americannursetoday.com/helping-new-nurses -set-priorities/

## Bibliography

Agency for Healthcare Research and Quality. (2004). Retrieved from http: //www.ahrq.gov/RESEARCH/jan04/0104RA25.htm

Arora, V., & Johnson, J. (2006). National patient safety goals: A model for building a standardized hand-off protocol. *Joint Commission Journal on Quality and Patient Safety, 32*(11), 646–655. doi:10.1016/s1553-7250(06) 32084-3

Rischer, K. (2015). How to help students set correct priorities in the clinical setting. *Keith RN Blog*, November 12. Retrieved from https://www .keithrn.com/2015/11/set-correct-priorities/

# 8

# The Value of Feedback

*Providing feedback to the preceptee, whether for performance improvement or to praise them, is essential for the growth and development of the nurse being precepted. For the purposes of this text, the term negative feedback will be avoided because no matter the form, feedback should be given so the person learns from the experience; therefore, the term performance improvement feedback will be used instead. Feedback can directly impact the preceptee for years, perhaps their entire career, so it must always be constructive. Feedback is forever. It is documented, recorded, referenced, and remembered for the lifetime of the nurse's career and beyond. Therefore, providing feedback should not be taken lightly and it should be done correctly. Providing feedback that is constructive, fosters learning, and assists in building the skill level and confidence of another is a skill that must be learned by the preceptor.*

After reading this chapter, the reader will be able to:

1. List the three main functions of feedback
2. List five items to remember when providing feedback
3. Define performance improvement feedback
4. Define the steps of the BEER method of feedback
5. List ways to provide positive feedback

# PROVIDING FEEDBACK

Nurses notoriously resist providing feedback for many reasons, including that they do not wish to be viewed as someone who criticizes their fellow professionals or students. Providing feedback is a learned skill and they have either been on the receiving end of poorly provided feedback or have provided feedback that was met with anger or ignored. Keep in mind that feedback has three main functions:

1. To reinforce positive behavior
2. To advise someone of a way to improve a behavior
3. To inspire the learner

Feedback is often confused with criticism, which is finding fault with people or things in a judgmental way.

## Poor Nurse Educators and Preceptors
- Criticize their preceptee
- Don't care about their preceptee or their success
- Focus on past mistakes

## Strong Nurse Educators and Preceptors
- Work with preceptees to identify what went wrong
- Take responsibility when needed
- Focus on making their preceptees better nurses
- Have a personal interest in their preceptees success and truly care about them
- Are focused on the future and how a mistake can be a learning experience
- Want the preceptee to learn from mistakes and move forward

## Negative Feedback

Negative feedback occurs when a preceptor (or other supervisor), patient, family member, or fellow staff member describes behavior or performance that requires improvement, but not specifically enough so positive changes can be made. No one can learn from this kind of negative, nonspecific feedback, so, ultimately, behavior and outcomes do not change.

### Positive Feedback

Positive feedback describes a behavior or performance that is welcomed, expected, and successful and should be repeated. Positive feedback reinforces desirable behavior or outcomes and helps to motivate learners. Unlike other feedback, positive feedback can be given in front of staff, patients, and families! Constructive, developmental, or performance improvement feedback is provided when a behavior or outcome is unsatisfactory and needs to be improved, but guidance for how to improve the behavior or outcome is also provided. "To be in an open, receiving state of mind . . . feedback must be positive, or at least guide the recipient to self-awareness and self-discovery" (Williams, 2011).

## DELIVERY OF FEEDBACK

Give feedback at correct times. The preceptor must judge what feedback can wait until the end of the clinical day and what feedback should be immediately provided (such as a current situation affecting patient safety). Do not just provide feedback at scheduled times (e.g., at the end of the day, or the end of preceptorship).

You should also be mindful of how people perceive you as a nurse. What is your relationship with the preceptee? What stage of the relationship are you in? For example, either the beginning of the relationship when you are still learning about each other or toward the end when the relationship is more established. In the beginning of the preceptor/preceptee relationship, the preceptee may be nervous and anxious, and any feedback may be perceived as criticism. Listed below are guidelines to follow when providing feedback to the preceptee:

### Don'ts

- Never give feedback when angry.
- Never provide constructive or performance improvement feedback in front of a patient, family, or other staff.
- Avoid using "judgment terms" in your feedback; these terms include words such as "good," "bad," "right," "wrong," "poorly," "incompletely," "incorrectly," "lazy," "always," and "never."
- Avoid starting sentences with the word "you" as such statements tell the preceptee they did something wrong, without providing

information on what led to your findings. In these situations, the preceptee may feel they are being attacked and consequently may become defensive. For example, "You need to change that dressing using better sterile technique" implies that sterile technique was not followed but does not tell the preceptee where the break in technique occurred.

- Avoid words such as "but," "however," and "although" in your feedback because they negate anything that came before them, whether positive or negative. For example, "You did a great job admitting that patient, but you forgot to ask about their current medications."
- Don't act arrogant or superior when interacting with the preceptee.
- Don't allow feedback sessions to interfere with patient care.

### Dos

Prepare before giving feedback.

- Address your concerns about the preceptee's performance specifically and immediately. If this is not possible, schedule a time when both you and the preceptee are available.
- Have a goal in mind before the encounter; know what you are trying to accomplish and what specific behaviors you are trying to change. If you don't have a goal for the conversation, it can deviate to other matters and the preceptee will feel that you are just criticizing them.
- Provide one-on-one feedback in a private setting. Consider also the potential "scariness" of that setting. A neutral area such as a staff room may be more comfortable to the preceptee, more conducive to learning, and less threatening than being summoned to the staff development or supervisor's office. Incorporate the building of critical thinking skills into your feedback. One method is to use open-ended questions and have the preceptee assess the situation and formulate an alternate means to discover and solve a problem. For example, if you notice a preceptee hanging an intravenous (IV) medication and observe that they correctly identify the patient but fail to introduce themselves, you might say: "Great job following the basic medication rights when administering the IV medication to Mrs. Smith. What could you have done that would have helped the patient recognize your role in her care?" Build critical thinking skills by sharing information, not by giving advice or saying how *you* would care for the patient

or what *you* would do. For example: "Your patient is scheduled for surgery at 0900. A dressing change, treatments, and several meds need to be given prior to leaving the unit. How are you going schedule your care?"

Be straightforward and objective.

- State your intention of providing feedback to the preceptee. This will disarm the situation and hopefully calm their nerves. The information you will be sharing is for learning purposes and the promotion of patient safety and quality of care.
- Be specific and direct with written and verbal feedback; don't "beat around the bush," but rather get to the point of the information to be conveyed. Briefly describe what you have directly observed. Not being direct causes confusion and frustration, exactly what you wish to avoid!
- Be objective in your description of what you observed (e.g., "your goals and documentation for your patients"). Descriptions must include who, what, when, and where. Start your comments with what you have seen, observed, or noticed, not what was "reported" to you.
- Focus on the preceptee's behavior, not their personality. Use adverbs that describe behavior the preceptee needs to focus on to change, rather than adjectives that describe their qualities. For example, it's better to say "Be specific in your injection site selection teaching with your diabetic patient" rather than "You always do a poor job teaching patients about their diabetes."

Make this into a teaching moment.

- Ask the preceptee to repeat back what directions they heard, if necessary, in order to correct any miscommunication.
- Ensure that the preceptee understands the rationale for actions.
- Build learning into the feedback. If you see that a preceptee consistently fails to follow correct procedures in providing care, have them review the literature or practice in the facility's nursing skills lab or with an educator. Consider the learning style of the preceptee when reviewing skills. At the next opportunity, have the preceptee verbalize the process with you and then perform the skill.
- Keep in mind the goal that you have both established and how your feedback will redirect the preceptee toward meeting that goal. For example, you may have determined that a goal may

be to complete a medication pass on an assignment of patients by week 3 of orientation. You observe that the preceptee is not meeting this goal. You share your observations (not prepared for medication pass in a timely manner and not being familiar with the medications to be given) with the preceptee.

- You can also pose observations in the form of open-ended questions which promotes critical thinking and involves the preceptee in a discussion rather than just listening to your observation. For example, you may say "I noticed you were hesitant when I asked you set up the IV pump for your patient. What are some of the questions you have regarding the setup?"

- If a potential error is caught, explain the consequences of the preceptee's actions. Give examples of how the action might have affected the patient. This will allow the preceptee to understand the impact that their action might have had on the patient and how it will affect the preceptee's future practice.

Be supportive.

- Give the preceptee the benefit of the doubt; they are not making mistakes in care on purpose. Always remember that first and foremost, you are an educator and that you are forming the future of this new nurse so be kind and compassionate. Be supportive at all times.

- Can the preceptee hear you? Stress and anxiety may cause the preceptee to not focus on or hear what you are telling them, either the directions before or the feedback (if an incident occurred) after.

- Allow the preceptee to respond to your feedback. Really listen to what they have to say. Maintain eye contact and remain silent; avoid interrupting. Encourage the preceptee to communicate with you by asking open-ended questions such as "Tell me what you are feeling right now?"

- Remember, even though you may be part of the unit staff, as a preceptor you are an advocate for the preceptee. Any issues the staff has with the preceptee should be handled with tact and care. How staff comments are handled can also affect the preceptee far into their career.

Be self-aware.

- Be aware of how *you* accept "feedback" or criticism. Accepting feedback, learning from it, and moving on is expected, but some people resent being corrected. Remember back to the last time you received unfavorable feedback and how it made you feel. Use that knowledge to guide you in providing feedback to your preceptee.

■ Accept shared responsibility if something went wrong in the care of the patient. Remember that your communication may have been at fault.

■ Have you considered what the benefits of providing feedback would be before you provide it? Will the preceptee learn and develop new skills or will they become angry and unable to function? If the preceptee is not being receptive and the issue is not a patient safety matter, it may be better to stop the interaction to allow the preceptee (and perhaps yourself) to calm down.

■ Consider your motives for providing feedback before providing it.Are you communicating information that you want the preceptee to learn? Or are you angry and trying to prove a point? Do you wish to help the preceptee and future patients? Or are you resentful?

Follow up on feedback.

■ Allow the preceptee time to consider what has occurred and what has been said, and to assist in formulating a plan of action so that the incident is avoided in the future. This will help to build their confidence levels.

■ Plan for a future opportunity when your preceptee can experience the same situation that they were unsuccessful in the first time and share this with them.

■ End the interaction on a positive and note and state how you will support the preceptee and continue to be present for them throughout the preceptorship, but ensure that they understand exactly what you are asking of them.

■ Document the encounter as required and notify faculty or staff development.

### Summary Thoughts on the Effective Delivery of Feedback to Preceptees

■ Preceptees appreciate feedback. They appreciated it as students in the clinical area and in their written work, and they appreciate it now, early in their careers. They should not be made to ask the preceptor for feedback; it should be provided willingly. Making them ask for feedback creates self-doubt in their performance and skills.

- There should not be more of one type of feedback than the other. For example, too much performance improvement feedback may cause the preceptee to doubt their chosen profession, leading to a snowball effect in which the preceptee feels they are "doing everything wrong." Conversely, too much positive feedback can cause the preceptee to not fully develop skills or critical thinking because of a feeling that they are already "doing everything right."
- Too much of either type will cause "feedback fatigue," resulting in neither type having the desired outcome.
- Lastly, be sure to keep careful notes on the preceptee's performance so you are not relying on memory alone.

### Fast Facts

If the preceptee has completely botched a situation, withhold immediate feedback because you may not be in the correct frame of mind to provide constructive feedback. Your comments could be fueled by anger, frustration, and disappointment, making your feedback harsh and critical, and providing no learning opportunity.

## "CONSTRUCTIVE" A.K.A PERFORMANCE IMPROVEMENT FEEDBACK

Providing constructive, or performance improvement, feedback is a definite skill and it is one that many administrators, nurse managers, supervisors, staff nurses, and preceptors do *not* have. Think back to your last performance appraisal. Did you benefit from the feedback? Have you improved your job performance based on the feedback? After the feedback was shared, did you feel positive—as if you had been given tools to succeed in the future—or were you upset and angry?

Performance improvement feedback should be given in the following situations:

- When it has been asked for
- When an error has occurred
- When patient safety is at risk

- When providing specific guidance
- As a follow-up to guidance or directions provided
- When correcting a situation
- When an error is repeated
- When the preceptee's work behavior does not meet expectations
- When conveying the consequences of poor performance

### Fast Facts

Performance improvement feedback should be given in such a way that the morale of the preceptee is not crushed so that they do not feel defeated in the new role.

Some additional guidelines on performance improvement feedback include the following:

- Performance improvement feedback should be given in person or over the phone if personal contact is not possible. Avoid giving this feedback through e-mail or in a text message.
- Always remember that you are an educator, so when providing performance improvement feedback, it should be considered as an opportunity for the growth of the preceptee.
- Instead of saying things like "you should have . . . ," "you shouldn't . . . ," or "next time don't . . . ," ask the preceptee what they could have done differently, how they could have handled a situation differently, or what could have been tried instead of what they did.
- Utilize your skills of empathy. Think back to when you were first beginning your nursing career and remember similar situations in which you found yourself. You might even share a story and what you learned from a similar situation.
- Listen, but avoid allowing the situation being discussed to turn into a "bitch" session. Guide the preceptee to solving difficulties encountered rather than placing blame on others. The preceptee may have a legitimate complaint regarding an issue on the unit. Help find a solution together.
- Monitor your body language. For example, sit rather than stand. Maintain eye contact. Do not cross your arms, tap your fingers, point at the preceptee, etc. Even though you should not provide

feedback when upset or angry, if you must respond quickly to a situation that has triggered such responses be sure your body language does not convey these feelings.

■ Note the preceptee may be angry with you after receiving feedback. Avoid behavior or words that could be considered retaliation against the preceptee. Be empathetic and understand it is not easy to take criticism.

■ Your attitude and words should communicate to the preceptee what you are expressing is important and that you are sincere.

■ Avoid performance improvement feedback based on hearsay or what was reported to you. Conduct your own investigation first, based on what was reported. Remember, feedback should be based on what you have observed directly. Your facts should be accurate. Give details, examples, and specific instances of the incident or problem.

■ Once the feedback is given, it is time to move on. Monitor the preceptee for attempts at learning from the experience and, when it is noted, provide immediate positive feedback.

## POSITIVE FEEDBACK

Lorenz, in her 2012 article, "Giving Positive Feedback to Nurses," notes that because nurses are literally taught to find out what is wrong with a patient (e.g., we assess a patient to discover what body system is not working, or their surroundings to ascertain what will cause harm), nurses often find it difficult to find things that are positive in order to relay positive feedback to preceptees and colleagues (not to mention family and friends). Similar to providing performance improvement feedback, however, it is a specific skill that can be learned. Demonstrating this skill to the preceptee will, we hope, ensure that it is passed on to others.

Some guidelines on providing positive feedback include the following:

■ Notice and acknowledge the positive actions of the preceptee, and say "thank you." This should also be said to all healthcare team members.

■ Actively seek out situations involving the preceptee that are going well. For example, "catch" the preceptee doing something correctly and praise them for it.

- Let your fellow staff and administrators know how much they are appreciated and why. It is okay to say that something someone does is appreciated, but also convey why it is appreciated. For example, "Thank you for completing that admission for me. I really appreciate it. It allowed me to help Mrs. Smith with her diabetic teaching."
- Voice appreciation for the action of the preceptee along with positive praise. Your message will be sincere and valued more.
- Even though you are providing positive feedback, you can include how the preceptee can change and evolve and progress in their career. For example, if the preceptee successfully inserted an IV line, review the steps necessary to become IV certified within your facility.
- For written feedback, be specific rather than general. For example, "Gave medication to five patients" could be better stated as "Accurately administered mediation to five patients utilizing the known rights of mediation administration and followed facility guidelines."

## FORGET THE SANDWICH AND HAVE A BEER!

Many managers and educators still use the "feedback sandwich" method of providing feedback, and you may have been a victim of this method as well. This method "sandwiches" constructive (i.e., "negative") feedback between two layers of positive feedback with the goal of softening the blow of any performance improvement issues. In reality, it only makes the giver of the less-than-positive feedback feel better about having to impart bad news and the receiver disappointed and stressed. The outcomes associated with this method of feedback are not always the most beneficial to the preceptee. For example:

- It is not straightforward or direct.
- It hinders the building of trust between the preceptor and the preceptee.
- The positive feedback is often forgotten because it is negated by the negative feedback.
- The importance of what action or behavior that needed to be improved is often lost.
- The preceptee's good action that should be repeated, which was shared in the positive portion of the feedback, is often lost after the negative behavior is verbalized.

**Fast Facts**

A better way to communicate the need for performance improvement or to deliver criticism is the BEER method. It summarizes the information in this chapter into a concise method.

- **B is for Behavior:** Communicate to the preceptee a specific undesirable behavior that has been directly observed. Use clear and concise language about what you find unacceptable; provide examples, including dates, times, and situations if possible. Do not generalize. Focus on behavior only, not personality (e.g., "The correct steps to ensure proper technique when suctioning the patient were not followed.").

- **E is for Effect:** Explain to the preceptee why the behavior is unacceptable. Explain how the unwanted behavior or action could potentially impact patient care and safety. Ensure that the preceptee understands what you are telling him or her (e.g., "What are the undesirable outcomes for the patient if the proper procedure for suctioning the patient is not followed?").

- **E is for Expectations:** Verbalize what you expect the preceptor to do. Very often the preceptee is aware that there is a problem but requires help to fix the situation. The preceptor as mentor is in a position to provide this helpful guidance. Involve the preceptee in creating a course of action to change their behavior, the end goal of which is not only to change the behavior but to build the confidence of the preceptee. In subsequent meetings with the preceptee, communicate what you have observed in the preceptee's movement toward eliminating or improving the undesirable behavior. Ensure that both you and the preceptee agree on the course of action.

- **R is for Results:** Explain how the changed behavior will positively impact patient care and safety, and cite examples. Also explain, if the behavior is not changed, what the implications will be (e.g., unsuccessful completion of nursing school or termination of a new employee if the behavior is severe). Continue to stress the main objectives of what the preceptee could do differently. Express confidence in the preceptee's ability to improve, and offer your continued support.

# WHAT IF THE PROBLEM IS PERSONALITY?

Remember back to your first job as a nurse or when you were a preceptee. One of the hardest skills to learn was how to get along with other members of the team. Nerves and anxiety can often induce behavioral issues in the preceptee, who is attempting to "fit in" while also attempting to impart to everyone that they are knowledgeable.

With this in mind, focus on the behavior! For example, suppose a preceptee continually leaves the unit for breaks without notifying staff. Personality-based feedback may focus on the fact that this is inconsiderate. Behavior-based feedback focuses on the fact that this places patients in danger and is against unit policy. For example, you might say, "I have noticed that you are leaving the unit for your break without notifying the charge nurse. When a staff member leaves the unit without notifying the charge nurse or covering nurse, it places the patients in danger because no one is monitoring them. What can you do to ensure that you are following the unit policy for patient coverage?"

## References

Lorenz, J. M. (2012). Giving positive feedback to nurses: Nurse managers can empower staff to advocate for quality care. *Advance Healthcare Network*. Retrieved from https://www.elitecme.com/resource-center/nursing/giving-positive-feedback-to-nurses/

Williams, R. (2011). Why "constructive feedback" doesn't improve performance. *Psychology Today*. Retrieved from https://financialpost.com/executive/why-constructive-feedback-doesnt-improve-employee-performance

# 9

# The Art of Delegation

*Patricia Yoder-Wise, in her book Leading and Managing in Nursing, noted that "Delegation is a complex, loophole-ridden, work-enhancing strategy. It can make the difference between caring for a group of patients and experiencing great anxiety and caring for that same group with a controlled expectation of what can be achieved. Used properly, delegation can enlarge the effect you have on patient care; used improperly, it can be frustrating and scary. Delegation is an art and a skill that can be developed and honed into one of the most effective professional management strategies any registered nurse can use" (Yoder-Wise, 2007). The nurse must understand that there is a difference between delegation and assignment.*

After reading this chapter, the reader will be able to:

1. List the five rights of delegation
2. List two points to remember regarding each right
3. Verbalize five points learned from the Joint Statement
4. List the four points that the registered nurse (RN) must be aware of regarding delegation
5. Discuss the decision tree for delegation

## DELEGATION POINTS TO REMEMBER

Delegation "is allowing a delegate to perform a specific nursing activity, skill, or procedure that is beyond the delegate's traditional role and not routinely performed. This applies to licensed nurses as well as UAP (unlicensed assistive personnel)" (National Council of State Boards of Nursing [NCSBN], 2016). Assignment is defined as the "routine care, activities and procedures that are within the authorized scope of practice of the RN or LPN/LVN or part of the routine functions of the UAP...it is included in the framework taught in the delegate's basic educational program" (NCSBN, 2016). Many nurses and other healthcare professionals are unaware of the process of delegation. This becomes evident when a preceptee is used as staff prior to the end of orientation, when competencies are not assessed prior to care, or when a member of the healthcare team is requested to perform a task not within their scope of practice.

Important points to remember regarding delegation are included in the statements of various nursing organizations:

- Accountability is central to delegation; ". . . since the nurse is accountable for the quality of nursing care given to patients, nurses are accountable for the assignment of nursing responsibilities to other nurses and the delegation of nursing care activities to other health care workers" (American Nurses Association [ANA], 2001, p. 17).
- Delegation involves "transferring to a competent individual the authority to perform a selected nursing task in a selected situation" (NCSBN & ANA, 2006).

Although there is great variation among the definitions of delegation, both The ANA and NCSBN define delegation as "the process for a nurse to direct another person to perform nursing tasks and activities" (NCSBN & ANA, 2006).

The ANA and the NCSBN both agree that:

- An RN can direct another individual to do something that that person would not normally be allowed to do.
- The RN retains accountability for the delegation.
- An assignment is defined as the distribution of work that each staff member is responsible for during a given work period.

- Supervision is the guidance and oversight of a delegated nursing task. Supervision could be either on-site supervision (ANA) or direct supervision (NCSBN), but both have to do with the physical presence and immediate availability of the supervising nurse.

If delegation is performed incorrectly, it can lead to decreased quality of care and unsafe patient conditions. Get organized; know what you need to know!

The NCSBN/ANA policy statement regarding delegation specifies:

- State nurse practice acts define the legal parameters for nursing practice. Most states authorize RNs to delegate (NCSBN & ANA, 2006). *Know the policy in your state.*
- The RN assigns or delegates tasks based on the needs and condition of the patient, potential for harm, stability of the patient's condition, complexity of the task, predictability of the outcomes, abilities of the staff to whom the task is delegated, and the context of other patient needs (NCSBN & ANA, 2006). *Be aware of the competency level of any staff member prior to assigning him or her to patient care.*
- All decisions related to delegation and assignments are based on the fundamental principles of protection of the health, safety, and welfare of the public (NCSBN & ANA, 2006).

Delegation, the preceptee, and the preceptor:

- Delegation is a skill that must be taught and practiced for nurses to be proficient in using it the delivery of care (NCSBN & ANA, 2006).
- Preceptorship should provide preceptees with opportunities to apply what they have learned. During this process the preceptee should be guided appropriately as to the process of delegation and supervision.
- For nurses to delegate effectively, they should have the experience to understand what it is they are delegating and the authority to delegate (NCSBN & ANA, 2006).
- Delegation skills are developed over time. Nursing employers need to recognize that a newly licensed nurse is a novice who is still acquiring foundational knowledge and skills (NCSBN & ANA, 2006).

**Fast Facts**

Although delegation is integral to preceptorship, the NCSBN/ANA Joint Statement on Delegation emphasizes that ". . . many nurses lack the knowledge, skill and confidence to delegate effectively so ongoing opportunities to enforce the theory and apply the principles of delegation is an essential part of *employment orientation and staff* development [emphasis added]" (NCSBN & ANA, 2006).

## THE FIVE RIGHTS OF DELEGATION

### Review with the Preceptee the Five Rights of Delegation

1. The right task
2. The right circumstance
3. The right person
4. The right communication and direction
5. The right supervision and evaluation

### Right Task

- Discuss with the preceptee what can or should be delegated.
- The task is within the job description of the team member.
- Are the tasks that they wish to delegate within the unit policies and procedures?
- The policies and procedures also review with the expected outcomes of the activity will be, the limits of the activity, and the competency training involved in carrying out the activity.

### Right Circumstance

- If assigning a task to UAP, ensure that the patient is stable and the outcome of the task is predictable.
- If the patient becomes unstable, the team member should know to communicate this to the RN for re-assessment of the patient.
- The right circumstance has the appropriate patient, setting, and available resources.
- Does the activity frequently recur among the patient population?

- Does the activity have a predictable outcome?
- Does the activity involve little or no modification from one patient or situation to another?
- Is the task free from requiring independent nursing judgment?

## Right Person

- Match the care to be performed to the right person (i.e., know the competencies of team members).
- Know the strengths and weaknesses of fellow healthcare team members prior to delegation.

## Right Communication and Direction

- The initial direction is the most important.
- There are five Cs of initial direction:
  - **Clear**: Does the team member understand what I'm saying?
  - **Concise**: Have I confused the direction by giving too much information?
  - **Correct**: Is the direction according to policy, job description, and the law?
  - **Complete**: Does the person to whom I'm delegating a task have all the information necessary to complete the task?
  - **Connect**: Follow up with the individual to assess the outcome of the task.
- Communicate specific details for each action.
  - List specific information that is to be collected, how it is to be collected, and when it is to be delivered; for example, "Get Mr. Jones's BP and report a BP greater than 130/80 to me right away."
  - List specific activities to be performed and any activity limitations.
  - List the expected results, potential complications, and when information should be reported to the nurse.
- The team member to whom a task is delegated must also communicate to the RN if they are unclear about the directions and task to be performed. They should seek to clarify what data should be collected (i.e. urine output, BP, etc.), how that data should be collected, when the data should be collected, and when the results should be reported to the RN. The RN should always seek to ensure that the team member understands the directions given and the task to be performed.

### Right Supervision and Evaluation

- Even after delegating a patient care task, the RN is responsible for monitoring the patient and the activity being performed.
- Follow-up should take place with the team member after the activity is performed.
- The patient should be assessed and evaluated for desirable and undesirable outcomes.
- The team member should have communicated any necessary patient information throughout the care given, and follow up on information provided.
- Be ready to assist the patient as needed.
- Document the care of the patient performed and outcomes measured.

### The Decision Tree for Delegation

The Joint Statement from the NCSBN/ANA includes a helpful decision tree that can be used in the first phase of delegation: assessment and planning (see Appendix B of the Joint Statement on Delegation here: https://www.ncsbn.org/Delegation_joint_statement_NCSBN-ANA.pdf). More information on delegation can be found at the organization's website: https://www.ncsbn.org/Delegation_joint_statement_NCSBN-ANA.pdf

### Step One: Assessment and Planning

*Goal: Give the Right Task Under the Right Circumstance to the Right Person*

While reviewing the delegation tree, keep in mind the following questions to better assign the care of the patient:

- What are the needs of the patient?
- What is the clinical condition of the patient?
- Is the level of decision making that will need to occur appropriate to the scope of practice of the person to whom I wish to delegate care?
- What level of assessment is needed?
- Is the outcome of the care and the patient's response to the care provided predictable?
- Is there a potential for adverse outcomes associated with the care?

- What are the cognitive and technical abilities needed to perform the activity, function, or task?
- Which member of the healthcare team has the needed scope of practice, required skill level, competencies, and experience to perform the task?
- What is the context of the situation and the environment? For example, was the patient just admitted? Is it a high-acuity environment?
- What level of interaction or communication is needed with the patient and with whom?

## Step Two: Communication

### Goal: Give the Right Direction

After the decision to delegate has been made, the next step is to communicate effectively.

- How is the skill or procedure to be accomplished?
- When and what information should be reported and to whom?
- What are the expected outcomes?
- How should the team member seek clarification about delegated care?
- If an emergency occurs during the care of the patient, how and to whom should the team member communicate?
- Is there anything special that this particular patient requires that may differ from patients having had a similar procedure in the past?
- Assess the team member's understanding of the procedure and the expected (and unexpected) outcomes.
- Be clear that you are available to direct and support.
- Ensure that the team member is willingly accepting the responsibility of what is being delegated to them.

## Step Three: Supervision

### Goal: Provide the Right Supervision

Even though care is delegated to another healthcare professional, the RN is responsible for the supervision and monitoring of the patient.

- What level of supervision and observation needs to be provided?
- How often should monitoring and observation take place?

- How will the RN verify that the care has been provided, completed, and documented?
- How will the team member or RN manage an unexpected change in the patient's condition?
- Be aware of the patient's current health status and stability.
- Can outcomes, responses to treatment, and risks be predicted?
- In what healthcare setting is care taking place (i.e., home, acute care, clinic)?
- What is the availability of healthcare resources and support for the patient and healthcare staff?
- How complex is the care being performed?
- The RN is at all times responsible for timely intervention and follow-up on any healthcare problems and concerns.
- The RN should be alert for subtle signs and symptoms and be proactive in the care of the patient before a patient's condition deteriorates.
- Be alert to any issues which will prevent the delegated care in taking place.
- Follow up with and evaluate the patient after delegated care is performed.

## Step Four: Observation and Feedback

### Goal: Assess the Effectiveness of Delegation

Once the delegated care has been performed, the RN is responsible for following up and ensuring that care was successfully and safely provided. This is the evaluation step and it is often forgotten in delegation.

- Was the delegation successful?
- Was the skill or procedure completed correctly?
- Was the desired patient outcome achieved?
- Was a better way to meet the needs of the patient discovered? Was this communicated to appropriate personnel?
- Is there a need to adjust the plan of care?
- Were there learning moments for staff or the nurse who delegated care?
- Was appropriate feedback and follow-up provided?
- Was positive feedback given when appropriate?

## CONSIDER THE FOLLOWING

NCSBN updated their delegation guidelines in 2015. They had two panels of experts who represented nursing education research and practice. The goal of the committee was to develop national guidelines based on current evidence-based practice to standardize delegation.

- Know the guidelines for delegation in your state.
- Delegation flows in the following direction: APRN to RN/LPN and UAP, RN to LPN and UAP, LPN when allowed by state to UAP.
- Delegation between same designations (i.e., RN to RN) is not "delegation" but a handoff because the staff involved have the same education.
- The healthcare facility must designate a nurse leader who is responsible for delineating care and to whom.
- The nurse leader must be part of a team of other nurse leaders that continually determines what responsibilities may be delegated and to whom.
- The healthcare facility must maintain delegation policies and procedures. These policies must also contain what cannot be delegated. These policies must be subject to frequent review and revision as needed and be consistent with Board of Nursing guidelines.
- The healthcare facility and nursing leaders must ensure that all nursing and UAP are educated regarding what responsibilities may be delegated.
- All healthcare workers must demonstrate competency on how to perform responsibilities that may be delegated to them.
- The nurse leaders are also responsible for reviewing the delegation process.
- The nurse leaders must maintain a positive culture within the facility that encourages delegation that follows the provided policies and procedures.

### References

American Nurses Association. (2001). *Code of ethics for nursing with interpretive statements*. Silver Spring, MD: Author.

National Council of State Boards of Nursing. (2016). National guidelines for nursing delegation. *Journal of Nursing Regulation, 7*(1), 5–14. doi:10.1016/S2155-8256(16)31035-3

National Council of State Boards of Nursing & American Nurses Association. (2006). *NSCBN and ANA issue joint statement on nursing delegation.* Retrieved from https://www.ncsbn.org/Delegation_joint_statement_NCSBN-ANA.pdf

Yoder-Wise, P. (2007). *Leading and managing in nursing* (4th ed.). St. Louis, MO: Mosby.

# 10

# Precepting the Accelerated BSN and Advanced Practice Registered Nurse (APRN)

*The basic concepts of preceptorship are the same across nursing. Yet there are subtle differences experienced in the role depending on the educational level of the preceptee. Standards of patient safety, critical thinking, and learning style are universal. However, each level of nursing education has its own particular concerns and the preceptee will enter the clinical area learning needs that require specialized support.*

After reading this chapter, the reader will be able to:

1. List five characteristics that set the accelerated BSN preceptee apart from their generic counterparts
2. List three issues that may present a challenge to the preceptor when precepting the accelerated BSN preceptee
3. List three things accelerated BSN preceptees require from faculty, preceptors, and educators
4. List 10 things a nurse must do to prepare to be an advanced practice nurse preceptor
5. List difficulties and barriers that the APRN preceptee encounters

## THE ACCELERATED RN TO BSN PRECEPTEE

The first Accelerated BSN program was developed at Auburn University nearly 30 years ago. That program and subsequent others were created to meet the needs of the nursing shortage. These programs have allowed adult students with previous degrees to quickly attain their RN/BSN and beyond.

### Fast Facts

The accelerated method of attaining a degree comes at the price of high attrition and even higher stress. Students find they are not able to complete the programs due to the pace, intensity, and oftentimes inability to meet financial obligations. Because of these factors, a comprehensive preceptorship is even more important.

Common findings of educators regarding accelerated BSN students and new nurses have been documented, but not many formal studies have taken place. What has been noted is that precepting and educating the accelerated BSN student can present a challenge due to many factors.

What sets this group of preceptees apart from the generic nursing preceptee or new nurse employee? The accelerated BSN preceptee is:

- More focused
- More successful and scores higher on NCLEX (National Council Licensure Examination for Registered Nurses)
- Highly motivated to learn and reach their goals
- Possessive of "real world" experience
- Goal oriented
- Organized
- Adept at the previously learned skills of research, use of databases and library resources, writing, and class preparation
- Able to work well within a group or cohort termed "cohort cohesions"
- Unafraid to speak aloud of experiences in clinical, class, or life settings
- More mature
- A passionate learner

Issues that may present a challenge to the preceptor when precepting the accelerated BSN student or new nurse:

- Educators and preceptors have voiced they find the accelerated preceptee "challenging" because the preceptees ask "why" and "why not" questions the preceptor or educator may not be prepared to answer.
- Preceptors may feel uneasy because the preceptee has a more diverse background than theirs.
- Requests that education be applied to real-world situations rather than memorization of facts.
- Preceptees may at first resent the close supervision of a preceptor as they are more independent and have functioned without supervision in previous positions.
- Preceptees may need assistance in developing coping and leadership skills because they may be viewed by their future nurse managers and healthcare facilities as having the background to become nurse leaders faster than their generic RN counterparts without the educational background to do so.

Accelerated BSN preceptees require the following from faculty, preceptors, and educators:

- Be aware of the background of the preceptee, and that they have home, family, and work responsibilities and obligations
- Be aware about how their life experiences will help them in their courses
- Be honest with the preceptee and tell them what they need to do to succeed
- Help them identify their learning needs
- Help them use their life and previous academic experiences to help them reach this new goal of becoming an RN
- Be aware of and share student assistance resources
- Focus on and teach only important information, nothing extraneous
- Review curriculum and course/clinical expectations prior to the start of a course or rotation
- Help them identify their strengths and how they can use those strengths to better themselves academically
- Provide with information on housing and financial management

What can schools of nursing and healthcare facilities can do to assist the accelerated BSN student and preceptee:

- Allow for social support and networking among the students both within the accelerated cohort and their counterparts in the traditional setting so that the students feel part of the school.
- Explanation prior to the clinical experience regarding the "rules" of preceptorship, including seeking supervision prior to performing a clinical skill. Oftentimes accelerated preceptees feel that they do not require such close supervision because of previous life experience.
- Communicate that respect of the preceptor by the preceptee is expected even when at times the preceptor may be younger than the preceptee.
- To be mindful of "surprise" schedule disruptions as the accelerated students are often caring for family and children and have schedules planned far in advance.
- Allow current students to interact and meet with graduates of the program so that current students can learn from someone who has "been through the process." Consider this also prior to admission acceptance, so prospective students can hear from current students or alumni.
- Be honest about the program rigor, how much time will be involved to complete coursework and clinical work, the intensity of the program, and that students may not be able to work while completing the program. The preceptor as well should be honest regarding the intensity and expectations of preceptorship.
- Provide budget and financial management information.
  - Give sources of additional financial resources such as scholarships, grants, and financial aid (school and government).
- Describe prior to student acceptance what a typical week in the program will entail.
- Personal therapeutic counseling resources and stress management for the preceptee.
- Mentor program with faculty, educator, and alumni participants.
- Provide refresher courses for writing, studying, test-taking strategies, and use of library databases.
- Understand that the accelerated nurse graduates may wish to quickly pursue a leadership position.

## THE ADVANCED PRACTICE RN (APRN) PRECEPTEE

Nurses who attain advanced degrees specialize in skills particular to one area of practice such as pediatrics or geriatrics. "By 2025, the nationwide projected shortage of primary care providers is expected to be between 46,000 and 95,000" (Hawkins, 2019). What does this mean for APRNs? It means there is an extraordinary opportunity for entry into the healthcare system. The competency assessment of those skills does not deviate between teaching facilities. Successfully acquired skills are documented using facility- or school-specific evaluation tools. Nurse practitioners seek to practice in a variety of settings, from acute care and ambulatory care to non-traditional settings and private practice.

The American Association of Colleges of Nursing (AACN) feels that nursing preceptors are a fundamental part of clinical learning for the APRN student. A properly formatted clinical learning experience provides the basis for creating a safe setting for the APRN student to gain valuable experience while developing clinical competence. According to the AACN, the APRN clinical preceptor functions "as a role model by incorporating evidence-based education best practices to ensure safe and effective patient outcomes." (AACN, 2020).

### Fast Facts

Precepting the APRN is no different than precepting the undergraduate nurse in many aspects. However, there are modifications that must be made to meet their specialized needs.

What is true with undergraduate preceptors is also true for those who precept the APRN; there is little in the way of recruitment, education, and retention efforts, or compensation.

Nurses who seek advanced degrees must be able to bring concepts learned in the classroom to the clinical area (theory into practice). They become, in many states, autonomous decision-makers in the care of patients. APRN faculty:

- Work together with the preceptor to create the clinical experience that will best meet the needs of the preceptee
- Are primarily responsible for ensuring program outcomes are met with regards to their institution's accreditation standards
- Are responsible for evaluating student outcomes, including the input of the triad of the faculty member, the student, and the preceptor

- Should evaluate the clinical setting to ensure it enables the goals of the clinical experience
- Ensure the APRN student learns the content and competencies specifically developed for the APRN and their focused population (family, geriatric, psychiatric, etc.)
- Need to clearly communicate the objectives of the clinical rotation to the preceptor

In summary, the APRN faculty has the responsibility of overseeing "the design, implementation, and evaluation of clinical practice experiences" that align "to student and program outcomes" (AACN, 2020).

All APRNs must be able to:

- Perform a complete health assessment as well as the competencies of their specialty
- Document a history and physical/assessment
- Analyze the data obtained from various sources (test results, etc.) to identify a patient care issue
- Select and prescribe (in some states) medication, treatments, and/ or alternative therapies to treat the patient
- Create plans of care that integrate other professions
- Utilize preventative healthcare measures
- Assist patients with identifying and utilizing community resources to meet their healthcare needs
- Work collaboratively with other healthcare professionals

The APRN preceptors should:

- Hold a license in the state where they are employed
- Hold a graduate degree from an accredited school of nursing and have at least a minimum of 2 years' experience as an advanced practice nurse
- Be assigned to the same unit or healthcare facility (i.e., clinic or other free-standing area) for at least 2 years
- Possess only a positive evaluation performance in the past year
- Ensure unit and facility-specific competencies and other annual education requirements are up to date
- Serve on either or both outside and facility professional development committees
- Analyze the setting where they wish to perform their preceptorship. Will it meet the needs of the preceptee? Will the preceptee be able to meet their learning objectives?

- Provide an orientation for the preceptee that includes communication of learning needs and other issues discussed in the chapter on organizing the clinical day
- Be realistic as to what might prevent the preceptee from meeting their objectives:
  - Non-supportive fellow staff or other healthcare professionals
  - Lack of learning opportunities
  - Objectives of the facility not meeting the goals of the preceptee
  - No opportunity for the preceptee to work independently
  - Pace of care too fast, making the preceptee focus on tasks to perform rather than learning the care they are to accomplish
- Be mindful as to what barriers exist on the unit or within the facility that would not allow the preceptee to integrate quickly and meet their learning objectives
- Be aware of time and frequency of site visits by the faculty. Be sure that these site visits work with both your schedule and that of the facility
- Make faculty are aware of any planned time off you have planned
- Attend planned meetings between the preceptee, the faculty, and yourself. Address any pressing issues and concerns immediately, but also share information at these planned meetings
- Be aware of the faculty's preferred means of communication (email, text)
- Work with faculty in order to provide a clinical experience that will meet the objectives of the course/clinical and advance the preceptees skills
- Allow the preceptee to be involved with the selection of patients that will assist them in meeting the course/clinical experience outcomes
- Allow the preceptee to work independently as much as possible after ascertaining they are a safe practitioner
  - However, too much autonomy must also be balanced with too much monitoring. Preceptees often feel because they are RNs, they are left alone to care for a patient without having the advanced clinical experience to do so.
- Utilize critical thinking concepts outlined in previous chapters
- Incorporate current clinical research data and evidence-based practice into clinical teaching
- Review or teach effective communication with the family, patient, and staff

- Demonstrate by example how to work collaboratively and communicate effectively with the healthcare team
- Allow the preceptee to work with and plan care with other members of the healthcare team
- Provide constructive, continual feedback, not just at midterm, at the end of clinical, or when asked by faculty
- Demonstrate by example the principles of healthcare resource utilization
- Review, as per school policy, the preceptee's clinical logs and other documentation to provide feedback as per the policy of the school
- Plan activities for downtime (such as in an free-standing facility and appointments with patients are canceled) either in simulated patient experiences or case study review
- Allow preceptee access to patient EMR as per facility policy. Be aware of the learning curve and time needed on the part of the preceptee in learning a new computer system
- Has contingency plans or an "assistant" preceptor that can assist if preceptor is off a day or has an unexpected absence

As nurses attain advanced degrees, APRNs also require a comprehensive preceptorship experience. However, this is not always the case. Difficulties and barriers that the preceptee encounter include:

- The requirement of their school to locate and secure their own preceptors and clinical placements
- Locating and retaining a preceptor because of the increased number of advanced practice nursing students but a limited amount of practice areas and nurse practitioners is also a concern. Schools of nursing may utilize their own educators as preceptors, medical students compete with APRN's for physician preceptors, and some healthcare facilities will not work with online nursing schools.
- Medical and physician assistant students may be given priority to preceptors over APRN students due to Medicare/Medicaid reimbursement issues
- Healthcare facilities may perceive APRN students as posing a "drag" on their healthcare providers because the student is taking them away from patient care or slowing the care provided
- Difficulty in acquiring advanced degree preceptors; schools of nursing and healthcare facilities may utilize preceptors that are inexperienced or not appropriate such as from a different profession

- Lack of faculty support for the preceptors
- Preceptors not being educated to precept advance practice nurses
- Inconsistent learning opportunities
- Having a patient care load so great that the preceptee was unable to take sufficient time with each patient in order to perform assessments or properly plan care
- Poor learning environments, lack of physical space because of the number of practitioners in a given space (i.e., MD office)
- Personal and family issues such as:
  - Financial burdens
  - Transportation
  - Child care
  - Work responsibilities
  - Lack of time to sufficiently prepare for the clinical experience
- Preceptor is not the specialty of the preceptee (i.e., Adult NP versus Pediatric NP) or the practice area does not meet the preceptee needs (i.e., preceptee is learning about health assessment, but is working with an NP in advanced care whose patients require advanced, not basic assessments)

Be aware that the NP may not be an experienced RN. There are RN to NP programs that allow a nurse to move from a traditional RN degree to NP practice without having had the clinical background usually thought of in an NP student. Be aware of the educational and clinical experience of the NP preceptee. Be mindful that the NP differs from the traditional nursing student in that they are acquiring advanced knowledge and skills beyond that of a registered nurse. Teaching and learning styles used for the traditional preceptee are still useful to the advanced practice student.

There has been some research conducted on the preceptees experience of preceptorship but very little from the perspective of the preceptor. Issues for the preceptor specific to the APRN experience include:

- Issues similar to undergraduate preceptors, including lack of compensation
- NP preceptees are ill-prepared for the clinical experiences, especially those who are in an RN to NP program and lack a strong clinical background
- Frequent inability to provide sufficient evaluation of the preceptee due to work demands and responsibilities on the preceptor

- Need for formal education in preceptorship
- Lack of support from the schools graduating the future nurse practitioners

## THE ONE-MINUTE PRECEPTOR MODEL

In Chapter 5, Critical Thinking Skills, it was noted that the One-Minute Preceptor Model (OMP) was not recommended for teaching the generic RN student or preceptee. However, the NP often has a physician for a preceptor due to the lack of sufficient specialty NPs. As of 2019, there was not standardized education for the NP preceptor and very often the NP student may encounter the "one-minute preceptor" model, so it is presented here.

The preceptor listens without interruption while the preceptee presents a patient case to them. When the preceptee finishes the presentation (which should include the history and physical and other significant data), the preceptor then asks five questions that encourage critical thinking:

1. **Get a commitment:** Ask the preceptee what they think is happening with the patient. What are some nursing diagnoses that are appropriate? What is their plan? What do they want to do for the patient? This begins interaction with the preceptee and preceptor.
2. **Probe for supporting evidence:** "What are issues have you considered for this patient?" "How did you rule things out or in?" Use questions that will assess the preceptees knowledge and critical thinking process. You can use this question to identify any gaps in knowledge—what do they know/not know and what can the preceptor teach them?
3. **Teach a general principle:** This can be about assessment findings, differential diagnosis, evaluation, recommended treatment, potential resources, and more. The preceptor should provide information based on any knowledge gap that was identified in the second step. Teaching a general principle is more effective than providing random facts. In this way, the preceptee can organize the information so that it is remembered for similar situations in the future.
4. **Reinforce what was done well:** Provide positive reinforcement.

5. **Give guidance about errors or omissions:** Provide feedback here with suggestions for improvement if needed.

## THE REASON FOR RIME

NP preceptors should not be quick to "write off" a preceptee who is not able to answer questions early on in the clinical experience. The preceptor should be ever mindful of the level of preceptee they are working with. Are they a first-year NP student or are they ready to graduate? Have they just graduated or are they an experienced NP just beginning a new position? The preceptee should only be held to the standard of the level of which they currently occupy, not to one above it, and certainly, not to one below. All preceptees can be considered a novice thinker/learner because they may be starting a new position in a different nursing specialty or just beginning their career.

The medical and dentistry fields use a tool called RIME (Reporter, Interpreter, Manager, and Educator) to help their preceptors guard against placing unreasonable expectations on new practitioners (MD, NP, and PA). Although there is not a plethora of research available on this method for nursing, it can be adapted to be used with the NP preceptee. This model identifies which level of performance that can be expected as a preceptee moves through a curriculum or clinical experience. The NP preceptee as well as the preceptor should be mindful of their progress and RIME provides a framework for feedback. The RIME tool can be found in Chapter 16, Preceptorship Competency Forms and Clinical Tools.

### Resources

The AACN has published a clinical preceptor resources guide for the APRN including tool kits and other essentials. Please see the *Resources* section at the end of the chapter. https://www.aacnnursing.org/Education -Resources/APRN-Education/APRN-Clinical-Preceptor-Resources -Guide

Another excellent guide to precepting students was published by Loyola University: "Precepting Graduate Students in the Clinical Setting" by Bette Case DiLeonardi and Meg Gulanick (2008), https://www.luc.edu/nursing /resources/preceptor/preceptormanualforpreceptinggraduatestudents/

## References

## AACN Essentials

American Association of Colleges of Nursing. (2020). *AACN essentials.* Retrieved from https://www.aacnnursing.org/Education-Resources/AACN-Essentials

Hawkins, M. D. (2019). Barriers to preceptor placement for nurse practitioner students. *Journal of Christian Nursing, 36*(1), 48–53. doi:10.1097/CNJ.0000000000000519

# 11

# Recognizing and Helping the Preceptee Who Is Struggling

*Many nurses have a "gut" feeling about the person they are pre-cepting. The preceptee may lack motivation in the form of self-directed learning or may not be socializing well with the rest of the healthcare team, or it may be that the preceptee "just doesn't get it." Gut feelings, however, cannot be the basis for evaluation or potential for dismissal from a nursing program or discontinu-ation of employment. The preceptor should have clear, concise guidelines for evaluating the preceptee, but very often the school, unit, facility, or faculty does not provide these guidelines. The following information will be helpful in evaluating and assisting both the preceptor and the preceptee in these situations.*

After reading this chapter, the reader will be able to:

1. List the steps to SUCCESS
2. List five warning signs that occur early in preceptorship that indi-cate a preceptee is struggling
3. Verbalize three open-ended questions that would assist the pre-ceptor in discovering why the preceptee is failing
4. List three items included in the "formula for success"
5. List what issues may cause a preceptee to struggle

## INITIAL OBSERVATIONS

Preceptors are usually quick to recognize, either by direct observation or monitoring, when a preceptee is struggling. They may also be forewarned by school faculty, staff development instructors, or fellow staff members. Once aware, preceptors should become more vigilant regarding patient safety and the monitoring of the preceptee. For example:

- Verify observations with faculty and staff development to ascertain if what is observed was either an isolated incident or a pattern of behavior.
- Promptly document and communicate any concern to staff development, unit manager, or nursing faculty in the case of the nursing student.
- Remain objective by focusing on the goals and clinical outcomes of preceptorship. It is not enough to report that you deem a preceptee as "unsafe" or that they are "just not getting it." Your observations must be based on the preceptee's failure to meet the written criteria of preceptorship.

## BEGIN AT THE BEGINNING

Evaluation of the preceptee should begin on the first clinical day and be an ongoing process. Preceptors should be clear about the expectations of the school, unit, facility, and themselves regarding the goals of preceptorship. The preceptor should:

- Review the goals and expectations of preceptorship as provided by the school or facility.
- Goals and expectations should be written up and signed by both the preceptor and preceptee and a copy provided to each. Copies should also be provided to the unit manager or faculty.
- Review all documentation provided by the school or staff development, including daily goal documentation and competency assessment.
- Review preceptee skill self-assessment and create clinical assignments based on learner needs as well as the needs of the unit or facility.
- Review their own expectations of preceptee behavior prior to the beginning of preceptorship.

### Fast Facts

Avoid "this is the way we do it here" thinking when reviewing skills and activities with the preceptee. As long as a preceptee can explain, using evidence-based practice, how to perform a skill or activity and it is safe, then acknowledge that there are different ways to assist the patient.

## IDENTIFYING THE PRECEPTEE WHO IS STRUGGLING

Marilyn Teeter, in her 2005 article, "Formula for Success: Addressing Unsatisfactory Clinical Performance," recommends a "formula for success" when addressing the unsatisfactory clinical performance of students. It uses the acronym SUCCESS to summarize seven steps in this process:

S—See it early.
U—Understand the student's point of view and feelings.
C—Clarify the situation with the student.
C—Contract with the student for success.
E—Evaluate the student's progress regularly.
S—Summarize the student's performance.
S—Sign the summary.

The recommendations that follow have been adapted from Teeter's article to provide a guide for the preceptor who is working with a struggling preceptee.

### Fast Facts

All areas of concern should also be addressed with the staff development educators, or with the faculty unit manager.

### See It Early

Note the following and document:

- Reporting late to work or to the clinical area
- Leaving the unit without permission or without telling staff

- Hesitation when providing answers to critical thinking questions
- Frequently asking for help without searching for the answer on their own
- Requesting that staff help with the assignment (beyond what would normally be required)
- Producing required paperwork that is sloppy or incomplete
- Exhibiting unprofessional behavior
- Being unprepared for the clinical day (e.g., not having basic supplies such as a pen or stethoscope)
- Being unsocial or distant with fellow staff
- Being easily distracted and not interested in the surroundings or in learning
- Being uneasy with clinical skills; making frequent mistakes
- Failing to review skills prior to performing them
- Stating that they are unclear about what the preceptor initially requested during follow-up to delegation

## Understand the Preceptee's Point of View and Feelings

Be sensitive to and empathetic about the preceptee's perspective. If you were in a similar situation, *how would you react*? Ask yourself the following questions and be honest in your responses:

- What would you be afraid of?
- How do you visualize what your role would be in a similar situation?
- Would you feel as if no one was available to assist you?
- Would you feel equipped to handle the situation?
- Would you recognize that there was a problem?
- What would be critical for you to focus on?

## Clarify the Situation with the Preceptee

Utilizing the model of preceptor behavior that was mentioned in Chapter 1, Preceptorship in a Nutshell, meet with the preceptee privately (not in front of staff, family, or patients). Be kind but objective and focus on behavior that has been directly observed. Normally, preceptors genuinely want preceptees to succeed. Attempt to gain insight into unwanted behavior by asking the preceptee the following therapeutic-style questions and allowing the preceptee appropriate time to respond:

- "Tell me how you feel while on the unit (or other clinical setting)?" (Is the preceptee comfortable or uncomfortable? Do they feel competent or incompetent?)

- "Share with me why you feel this way."
- "Tell me how you feel when you are working with your patients" (e.g., good, happy, sad, useless, upset, etc.).
- "Are you happy with your work as a student nurse or nurse?"
- "Are you happy about being a nurse or becoming a nurse?"
- "Tell me where you see yourself in a few years" (e.g., this type of setting, this unit, this career).
- "Tell me what you feel you are having difficulty with during work or clinical" (e.g., the work, the setting, the skills, fellow staff, expectations, etc.).
- "In your words, why do you feel this is causing difficulty?"
- "Share with me how you feel you are doing. How would you evaluate your performance?"
  - If the preceptee is a student, be aware of their semester level (e.g., freshman versus senior), expected knowledge level, and previous clinical performance.
  - Be aware of patterns of behavior rather than isolated incidents.
  - Be aware of the level of risk to the patient that has occurred (minor versus serious).
  - Gently interject your personal observations and honest evaluation.
  - Provide clear, specific examples of any safety or quality-of-care issues.
  - Document any measures that were undertaken to address the situation.
  - Staff development and nursing faculty depend on the documentation that preceptors provide. Be sure that it follows facility guidelines and is complete.
- "What do you think you need to do to be successful?" At this point you can identify and clarify what the preceptee must objectively do to be successful (e.g., passing clinical, completing preceptorship).

### Contract with the Preceptee for Success

While reviewing the above questions with the preceptee, encourage them to take notes and document points that both of you feel are important regarding objective observations. Some guidelines for contracting with the preceptee follow:

- Both the preceptor and preceptee should sign the notes.
- The notes should be referred to as a "formula for success" (Teeter, 2005) and should:
  - Be objective and focus on behaviors.
  - Focus on the potential for success not failure.

- Use positive, not negative, wording.
- Use encouraging, not discouraging, wording.
- Be clearly worded, legible, and understandable.
- Include what the preceptee has stated and what resources they would need to successfully meet the objectives. Assist the preceptee with ideas and suggestions.
- Document on the "formula for success" that, in order to meet the objectives, a pattern of successfully meeting the objectives must be observed. It is not enough to be successful in an objective just once.
- Document that the preceptee must meet all other clinical objectives while also focusing on the areas in which they have previously been unsuccessful.
- Include a time frame for meeting to discuss the "formula for success" objectives.

- Based on the performance and degree of severity of the infraction, the preceptor can recommend many courses of action to assist the preceptee, among them:
    - Extra coaching and assistance with clinical preparation
        - A "re-grouping" with the preceptor (e.g., the preceptee may need to begin preceptorship again with review of the basics that were explained at the start)
        - Allowing the preceptee time to review all patient care documentation
        - Decreasing the patient assignment number and acuity
        - Taking over the skill for the preceptee, closely monitoring, and only allowing the preceptee to repeat the skill after remediation and close observation
        - Gradually letting the preceptee attain independence again after they are evaluated and deemed to be safe
    - Time in a skills or simulation lab
    - Change of unit (confer with nursing faculty and staff development prior to making this suggestion to assure that there is the possibility for change of venue)
    - Change of preceptor (see Chapter 13, Conflict Resolution and Bullying in Nursing for approaches to preceptor–preceptee conflict)
- Emphasize with the preceptee that they will be successful if the guidelines contained in the notes are followed.
- Keep a copy of the notes, and advise the preceptee to do so as well.
- Notify the unit manager and staff development of your conversation with the preceptee.

- If an infraction was severe, nursing faculty, staff development, and the unit manager should be notified immediately. The continuation of the preceptorship may need to be decided with input of the preceptor.
- Many preceptors weigh the severity and frequency of the infraction in their decision to notify faculty or staff development. If the infraction is minor and has occurred only once, the preceptor may choose to handle the remediation on their own but should still communicate to faculty, unit manager, and staff development. This is recommended so that guidance and suggestions can be obtained and to keep everyone "in the loop." If, however, the infraction was severe or the preceptee commits the same error again after evaluation by the preceptor, then it is imperative that all concerned be immediately notified and a course of action planned.

### Evaluate the Preceptee Regularly

As a preceptor, there are scheduled times that you must meet with the preceptee to evaluate progress. The number of meeting times should increase with the preceptee who is experiencing difficulty.

- Evaluate often to redirect the preceptee toward the mutually agreed upon goals if necessary.
- Each evaluation session should be documented; note details such as supportive measures and learning opportunities provided. This type of documentation supports the preceptor and the preceptee and protects both from unfair decisions.
- Refer to the "formula for success" in your discussions.
- Be sure to address the successes you have observed and share these with the preceptee. Evaluation meetings should not only address concerns.
- Patiently and clearly identify where improvements still need to occur.
- Document as per facility guidelines.
- Have the preceptee make additional notes on the "formula for success" and provide a new copy for the preceptee and for your files.
- Continue to emphasize that by following the "formula for success" the preceptee will indeed be successful in preceptorship.
- Sign and date any updates to the "formula."

## Summarize the Preceptee's Performance

At the end of preceptorship, the preceptee's performance is evaluated and summarized. This could be at the end of the clinical period, at the end of the facility-specified orientation period, or at an agreed-upon time period for a continually unsuccessful new employee. The following considerations should be incorporated in evaluating and summarizing the preceptee's performance:

- Be objective and use behavioral terms.
- Include the preceptee's perspectives.
- Determine whether the preceptee has attained the stated and agreed-upon goals of the preceptorship.

### The Bottom Line

When preceptorship has concluded, the preceptor must review the outcome and conclude if the struggling new nurse or student has successfully met the objectives. The following questions will help you to ascertain if the preceptor has been successful:

- Did the preceptee change their behavior so it now meets the clinical objectives?
- Are the preceptee's clinical skills meeting acceptable standards or are they below standard?
- Did the preceptee change their behavior but is performance still consistently below standard?
- Is the preceptee a safe practitioner able to provide high-quality, patient-centered care? Do you trust the preceptee to care for patients in a safe manner?

If you feel that the preceptee has been *successful* in meeting the objectives of preceptorship, then sign off as such on all school or facility documentation. In addition:

- Praise the preceptee in being able to meet the objectives and goals and wish them continued success.
- Complete all facility- or school-required documentation and communicate all findings with the staff development or school faculty member.

If the preceptee was *unsuccessful*, then assist them in realizing that the behavior has not changed and they have not successfully met objectives.

- Refer to the "formula for success" and identify where there are still weaknesses.
- Remember that as a preceptor, you also should be a mentor, and this process does not come to an end if the preceptee has not been successful. The preceptee may have failed at this particular goal, but they are not a "failure" and should not be made to feel this way. The preceptor can still provide guidance as to the next steps the nurse preceptee may take. These include offering the following suggestions:
  - "You need more time to improve your clinical skills. Repeating the semester would give you a chance to perfect those skills that need some work."
  - If the preceptee is a student, then suggest remediation back to the simulation lab at their school: "This will give you a chance to develop your skills in a less stressful environment."
  - "Due to all the stress and responsibilities in your life right now, this may not be the right time for you."
  - "You are so good with people [if that is the case]. Perhaps nursing may not be the right career choice for you, but a career working with people is still a good fit." (Expand on this, noting the preceptee's people skills.)
  - "This may not be the clinical area for you. Have you considered _____ type of nursing?" (If a preceptee is not successful in a hospital setting, they may find more job satisfaction in a less acute area such as long-term care or home care).

If the preceptee has changed their behavior but is still *performing inconsistently*, this needs to be documented and communicated to staff development or nursing faculty.

- If possible, request additional time to work with the preceptee to improve a specific area. Document appropriately.
- If a skill still needs improvement, the preceptor can recommend remediation to the simulation or clinical skills lab. Document appropriately.
- If, after objective review of the skill, the preceptee has made improvement sufficient to meet objectives, then proceed with documentation of successful completion of preceptorship. Communicate your findings and document appropriately.
- If, after education and remediation, the preceptee is still unsuccessful, communicate your findings to staff development and nursing faculty and document appropriately.

**Fast Facts**

Some preceptors and educators unknowingly set up the preceptee to fail. A new preceptor may forget what it is like to be a novice or student nurse, or they themselves have received no guidance.

## DID YOU SET THEM UP TO FAIL?

Preceptors may be unaware of what the student is currently studying or what the objectives of the clinical experience are and therefore set the preceptee up to fail. Avoid this by:

- Assigning patients to the preceptee that reflect what the preceptee is learning in their courses
- Being sure you are clear as to the objectives of clinical, question faculty if you are unsure of what patient assignments would be appropriate
- If your preceptee is a new nurse, select a less complicated patient at the beginning
- Avoiding thoughts of "they can do it if they try," "I had to do this so they do to," "this is the way we've always done this"
- Knowing that the preceptee does not learn by just watching you perform a task
- Avoiding overloading the preceptee with too much information all at once
- Avoiding sharing information when the preceptee is particularly anxious, they will not remember
- Encouraging the preceptee to ask questions. They are unsafe if they "assume" to know the answer or how to perform a task
- Being open to the preceptee telling you if they made a mistake. Mistakes can be valuable learning experiences, not an opportunity for punishment

### Sign the Summary/Evaluation

In the case of a facility preceptorship, complete and sign all required documentation indicating that the preceptee has successfully completed preceptorship.

## Reference

Teeter, M. M. (2005). Formula for success: Addressing unsatisfactory clinical performance. *Nurse Educator, 30*(3), 91–92. Retrieved from http://preceptor .healthprofessions.dal.ca/?page_id=337rse

## Bibliography

Docherty, A. (2018). Failing to fail in undergraduate nursing. Understanding the phenomenon. *Nursing Education Perspectives, 39*(6), 335–342. doi:10.1097/01.nep.0000000000000350

# The Unsafe Preceptee and How to Avoid "Failure to Fail"

*Preceptors often feel pressure from staff development, unit managers, or facility administrators to successfully pass a preceptee through preceptorship even when the preceptee has not met the clinical objectives or is someone whom the preceptor may consider "unsafe." It is sometimes conveyed to preceptors (and staff development educators) that adding the new nurse to the facility would increase staffing levels, and if they are not allowed to pass, staffing levels will continue to be negatively affected, decreasing employee morale and continuing to adversely affect staffing levels. Therefore, careful documentation supporting the progress, or lack thereof, of the preceptee is very important as is supporting the preceptor throughout the process. As a preceptor, you have probably experienced a student who you felt was not safe, or who just "didn't get it." You probably wondered "how did they make it this far?" and wondered why they had not been excused from their nursing program before they reached your clinical area. You have therefore experienced "failure to fail."*

After reading this chapter, the reader will be able to:

1. List five factors that contribute to failure to fail
2. List three factors that describe unsafe practice

**3.** List five things to consider when objectively documenting on the preceptee

**4.** Explain how the SUCCESS method can be utilized to document

**5.** List three ways to prevent unsafe practice in a preceptee

## WHY DO EDUCATORS AND PRECEPTORS "FAIL TO FAIL"?

Although preceptors should never be solely responsible for firing a new staff nurse or the failure of a nursing student, they do contribute, along with the clinical educator and faculty associates, to the phenomena known as "failure to fail." Why do they do this? Because:

- They don't feel confident addressing a potential "failure" moment with the preceptee.
- They feel that *they* would be thought of as a failure by fellow staff.
- The placement of a student within a nursing program, such as a first-year student versus a student at the end of the program. If the student has just started, then the preceptor may feel the preceptee "hasn't had a chance." If they are toward the end of the program, the preceptor may feel it is too late (time and money spent factor).
- They lack clear clinical objectives.
- They have a personal bias toward the student or nurse.
- They fear litigation.
- They fear reprisal from management (that they are causing a "lack of staffing").
- They are unsure of what or how to document and to whose attention it should be brought.
- They have an attitude that a preceptee is "good enough" if they are nominally competent but not a strong nurse, and that maybe they will improve given time.
- They feel that the preceptee might be "ok somewhere else, but not on this unit."
- They hope that a preceptee will fail in some other area so that the burden of contributing to their failure or removal from a unit will not fall on them.
- They are pressured to pass the preceptee to increase staffing levels or maintain school quotas.
- They fear poor faculty or preceptee evaluations.

Preceptors should rightfully feel they are the gatekeeper between the preceptee, the safety of the patients, and the healthcare system as a whole. But without clear cut guidelines how can a preceptor determine if a preceptee is safe? Very little exists in the literature to guide a preceptor. Vague recommendations note if a student is unsafe, unprofessional, unethical, lacking in knowledge, lacking awareness of a patient problem and addressing it and/or failing to seek help from staff/educator/preceptor then they can be deemed as making "unsatisfactory progress." Is a preceptee unsafe because of one infraction or multiple? It is universally felt that a solution as to how to cope with the unsafe student is not known, however, once decided upon it should be exclusive to each school or facility.

## Fast Facts

The preceptor who takes patient safety seriously must reflect at all times on the question, "Is this preceptee safe? Are they providing safe patient care?" If the answer is "no," then the decision to document and notify the appropriate faculty or staff personnel is justified.

No one study has been completed that can unequivocally say "this is an example of an unsafe preceptee and this is what you do about them." However, a major theme across all research into unsafe students and nurses is that of *context and patterns* (Tanicala, Scheffer, & Roberts, 2011) with an overarching theme of patient safety.

For example, a first semester or first-year student should not be held to the same standards as a senior student or graduate nurse. Preceptees can only be held to the standards they have been taught. All students and preceptees *are* held to the competencies they learned for the unit or the course. One error may not be considered unsafe practice, but patterns of the same type of error are. A preceptee who cannot perform a skill correctly once may not be considered unsafe, but a preceptee's inability to perform a skill correctly after multiple attempts and after remediation is another matter. Any violation of patient safety is an automatic issue.

The preceptor must document as per facility or school guidelines any infraction or patient safety violation that is objectively observed. Notify appropriate facility and/or school personnel as per policy. Do not wait until the end of the preceptorship experience to notify the appropriate parties as this is a disservice to both the preceptee and the patients. First, the preceptee will not have the opportunity to learn from a mistake, and second, patients may also be placed in further danger.

## WHAT DEFINES AN UNSAFE PRECEPTEE?

Being an unsafe nurse can mean different things to different educators and preceptors. However, the following guidelines with examples can be followed:

- Unsafe clinical practice
  - Specific patient safety issues such as failure to correctly identify a patient or failure to utilize the correct method of medication administration
  - Failure to communicate patient findings or care provided to fellow healthcare personnel despite being reminded to do so
  - Poor critical thinking skills
  - Not following instructions
  - Overconfidence (leads to not seeking assistance or verbalizing lack of knowledge)
  - Defensive attitude
  - Does not follow standard procedures correctly or unit/facility policies and procedures (i.e., hand washing, HIPPA, documentation)
  - Not prepared to care for a patient—research on patient such as disease process, medications to be administered, care to complete is insufficient or not completed
- Unprofessional behavior
  - Inappropriate behavior toward a patient
  - Uncaring behavior toward a patient
  - Lack of cultural sensitivity
- Unethical behavior
  - Failure to document
  - Falsifying documents
  - Lying (such as assessment data or patient findings)
  - Plagiarism
  - Hiding mistakes and/or not verbalizing errors
  - Not "owning up" to errors
  - Verbal/physical abuse of a patient
  - Unaware of their scope of practice and may be practicing above it

- Knowledge deficit
  - Failure to recognize actions, side effects, and safe/unsafe parameters of medication
  - Inability to apply learned knowledge to current patient event
  - Failure to move from theory to practice
- Failure to seek assistance when needed or when patient care warrants
- Failure to recognize when a patient is in distress or other patient care difficulty

The following may be thought of as a preceptee displaying unsafe practices, but removed from the critical situation, can display a student who requires additional education or remediation. This can include:

- A preceptee who makes independent care decisions without consultation with the preceptor (very often these decisions are incorrect)
- Being uncomfortable in performing a learned skill (not appropriate for a new skill)
- Poor documentation—data not complete
- Failure to verbalize observed patient issues or change in condition
- Not prepared to take care of a patient (despite being provided with clear guidelines as to how and what to prepare)
- Does not respect the needs or requests of the patient
- Disorganized
- Late to the clinical area

The importance of being objective cannot be overemphasized. Preceptors should avoid hearsay and only document or comment on what is directly observed. To maintain objectivity, consider the following:

- Did what occur present a patient safety issue?
- Was what occurred a misunderstanding on your part? On the part of the preceptee?
- Did a miscommunication take place among staff or between the preceptor and the preceptee?
- Did what occur contribute to a pattern? Has it happened before?
- What was happening with the preceptee at the time of the issue? Were they ill, stressed, did they not understand what they were supposed to do? Remember, if you have created an environment of safety, the preceptee should feel free to discuss any underlying issues with you. Be sure that the preceptee knows what is expected

of them. Guide them to any assistance they may require (stress reduction, health concerns).

- Does the preceptee have a personal issue that is interfering with their learning? Does their behavior interfere with learning and staff interaction with them? If so, speak to staff development or the preceptee's clinical educator
- If an objective conclusion cannot be attained, consider having another preceptor work with the preceptee. Are their conclusions similar?

**Fast Facts**

Preceptors should *never* be *solely* responsible for the hiring and firing of new personnel or the failure of a student. Your role is to provide your objective opinion as to the progress or lack thereof and to consult with appropriate personnel as to your concerns.

Clear policies and procedures both within a healthcare facility and a school of nursing are necessary to assist faculty, clinical educators, and preceptors in recognizing and dealing with unsafe students and nurses. These policies and procedures should be objective and have measurable parameters and guidelines to assist in the evaluation of a preceptee.

## A QUESTION OF ETHICS AND MORAL REASONING

In the research regarding what constitutes a safe vs unsafe preceptee, there was strong agreement that the most unsafe incident a preceptee or practicing nurse can commit is to cover up a patient care mistake or error. This is a clear violation of the American Nurses Association (ANA) Code of Ethics Provision 3.4, which states that in the event of an error or a near miss, nurses must adhere to their respective institutional guidelines when "reporting such events to the appropriate authority...nurses may neither participate in, nor condone through silence, any attempts to conceal the error" (ANA, 2014).

Ethical standards should guide educators and preceptors to discern if a preceptee is following safe practices. The difficulty is that not all preceptees have strong ethical or moral backgrounds and those subjects are beyond the scope of a school of nursing or preceptor to teach in isolation. Ethical considerations in patient care and the importance of ethics with regards to patient safety should be emphasized throughout basic nursing curriculum. Moral reasoning is difficult to teach as it is shaped by the preceptees background and attitude. Merely teaching ethical standards does not guarantee that a preceptee will follow them. Understanding how a violation of them endangers patients may not influence a preceptee. Teaching morals and ethics in basic nursing education is difficult because of the following issues with the preceptee:

- Fear of failure
- Lack of understanding
- Lack of knowledge of nursing's professional standards
- Lack of clear guidelines in basic nursing education (what is ethical and moral?)
- Lack of ability to verbalize limits in professional practice due to lack of knowledge of standards

## "TEACHING" ETHICS

Teaching ethics and morals may be beyond the scope of a school of nursing's curriculum. Educators and preceptors can model at all times, however, accountability, honesty, maintenance of professional standards, trust, respect, critical thinking, moral standards, and safe practice to influence these standards in their preceptees.

## HOW TO PREVENT UNSAFE PRACTICE

Preceptors have an opportunity to prevent unsafe practice. The most important aspect of preventing unsafe practice is to provide a safe learning environment where communication between the preceptee and preceptor is expected and encouraged. Effective communication is seen as the number one preventative measure to unsafe practice. Other measures include:

- Have a clear understanding of the objectives of a course (for a student preceptee) or of the unit orientation (in the case of a new nurse).

- Share with the preceptee a clear set of expectations of the preceptor. This can include the care to be given and what should be communicated to the preceptor concerning patient care.
- Encourage the preceptee to "ask before doing" and to make the preceptor aware of anticipated care.
- Question the preceptee prior to the start of preceptorship as to their expectations of the preceptorship experience. In this way the preceptor will learn of unrealistic goals and expectations of the preceptee. The preceptor can take this information and formulate, along with the preceptee, realistic learning goals.

## WHAT TO DO IF A PRECEPTEE IS "UNSAFE"

Once identified either through direct observation or report by educators or faculty, the preceptor must develop a plan of action. Most importantly, the preceptee is to be more closely monitored than before to ensure patient safety. At all times, the preceptor is judging whether the incident was a major or minor concern. Minor concerns can be addressed between the preceptor and the preceptee. Major patient safety issues require the following measures:

- If an incident occurs while the preceptor is observing, stop the preceptee immediately and take over the skill that they were performing. Do not reprimand the preceptee in front of patient, family, or other staff.
- Confer with staff development or clinical instructor to ascertain if the observed behavior/incident was isolated or part of a larger pattern. Again, judgment must be utilized as to major vs minor occurrence or if the issue was seen a second time after preceptee/ preceptor communication.
- Judge who should participate in remediation for the preceptee prior to speaking to the preceptee so assistance can be offered. For example, should the preceptee participate in remediation in a school or facility simulation lab? Should the preceptee review written policies?
- Speak with the preceptee directly as to the observed issue. Question the preceptee if they were aware of the incident and if they have any insight into why the incident occurred.
- The incident should always be used as a learning opportunity, but the preceptee may not acknowledge that the incident was a patient safety issue.

- Allow the student to assist in the development of a plan of action.
  - Several tools have been developed, such as the SUCCESS method (see Chapter 11, Recognizing and Helping the Preceptee Who Is Struggling), to guide the preceptor and preceptee in understanding what is to be accomplished and how it will be measured.
  - Other documentation options include utilizing the charting method of SOAP (Subjective, Objective, Assessment, and Plan) to organize a difficult learning situation and to ascertain if the preceptee is successful in meeting a measurable goal.
  - Yet another model used with dentistry students, but easily adaptable to nursing, is that of PET (Prime, Partition, Praise, Empathy and Teach). See Chapter 16, Preceptorship Competency Forms and Clinical Tools.
  - Be specific in what the preceptee needs to accomplish to be deemed safe in their practice. What should they practice? Where should they practice? How will they be remediated? Will there be a test prior to the preceptee returning to the unit? What tools will be used to determine competence? By when should competency be accomplished?
- Notify staff development, unit manager, clinical educator etc. as to the observed behavior or incident that occurred.
- Document objective findings per school or facility guidelines.
- When in doubt, seek out the assistance of a more experienced preceptor or clinical educator. This will assist the preceptor in maintaining objectivity. Confirm with them what you feel you have observed.

## "AN OUNCE OF PREVENTION"

All preceptors and educators should correctly anticipate that a patient care error will occur, and therefore use some activities to prevent unsafe practice.

- Demonstrate a new skill first and have the preceptee return demonstrate in a safe environment.
- Always observe the preceptee with a new skill until competency has been achieved.
- Encourage the preceptee to practice a new skill until they achieve mastery.

- Have the preceptee read about the skill they will be performing, either their school texts in the case of a student preceptee or unit procedure material.
- Question the preceptee prior to the skill being performed, utilizing critical thinking skill builders.
- Create a non-punitive environment so a preceptee feels comfortable approaching the preceptor with concerns or if a mistake or error has occurred.
- Provide feedback immediately in private when an error or unsafe issue has occurred. Be specific and objective.
- Allow for differences in practice. Acknowledge that a preceptee may have learned a skill differently. As long as the preceptee can verbalize evidence-based practice for why they are performing a skill as they are and they do so in a safe manner, then allow for alternative ways to complete care.
- Do not lower standards to fit those preceptees who are not performing as they should.
- Always use errors or mistakes as a learning tool. Use them in education of future preceptees and consider how they can be avoided in the future.
- Preceptors learn from errors as well… how can they be prevented?

### Fast Facts

No matter the methods used, it should be noted that the primary purpose of a preceptor is to TEACH so if a preceptee is having difficulty, they are not to be "written off" as "not getting it" or "not fitting in." All efforts should be made to assist the preceptee in identifying areas that require improvement, developing a method to address the situation and objectively measuring the outcome.

If at all possible, the preceptor *should not* be part of the termination process of a new nurse employee or of a failed student.

- Preceptors should not be solely responsible for assigning failing grades or recommending termination.
- Unfortunately, many facilities use the preceptor as the person to deliver the bad news that the new employee is being terminated for unsuccessful preceptorship. This should not be allowed to

occur because the preceptor is, by definition, is the person at the facility who is viewed as being there to assist new nurses and students. For this reason, the preceptor should not be the one to terminate employment or completion of nursing school.

## References

American Nurses Association. (2014). *Code of ethics for nurses*. Retrieved from https://www.nursingworld.org/coe-view-only

Tanicala, M., Scheffer, B., & Roberts, M. (2011). Pass/fail nursing student clinical behaviors phase I: Moving toward a culture of safety. *Nursing Education Research, 32*(3), 155–161. doi:10.5480/1536-5026-32.3.155

## Bibliography

Docherty, A. (2018). Failing to fail in undergraduate nursing. Understanding the phenomenon. *Nursing Education Perspectives, 39*(6), 335–342. doi:10.1097/01.nep.0000000000000350

# III

# Preparing the Preceptee for the Future

# 13

# Conflict Resolution and Bullying in Nursing

*Conflict and bullying occur among all people and in all professions. This is true for many reasons: psychological, cultural, and biological. It appears, however, that they occur more frequently in the nursing profession than in any other. Preceptors need to teach preceptees how to effectively manage conflict and bullying during preceptorship because safe, quality care involves communication, trust, and cooperation with fellow team members. Remember, too, that the preceptor models the example for professional behavior that the preceptee will follow.*

After reading this chapter, the reader will be able to:

1. Define conflict
2. List the causes of conflict
3. List the causes of bullying
4. Verbalize how to resolve conflict
5. Verbalize how to deal with bullying

## DEFINITION OF CONFLICT

According to Conerly (as cited in Hiemer, 2011), conflict can "occur at any time and in any place, originating between two individuals or groups when there is a disagreement or difference in their values, attitudes, needs, or expectations." It can also occur as a result of miscommunication and lack of information. At some point while at work, nearly everyone experiences indecision, anger, stress, or disagreement with coworkers. While this may be caused by conflict, it is not conflict in and of itself. A situation meets the definition of conflict if:

- Two sides (people, parties, groups, teams, etc.) need something from each other and without the item, they are at risk.
- Each side blames the other for causing the difficulty.
- Each side displays its anger either overtly or covertly, hiding it behind politeness and civility.

Additionally, in nursing conflicts, the behavior of the two sides causes problems that affect patient outcomes and safety, unit cohesiveness, job performance, staff morale, and staffing levels.

## NOT ALL CONFLICT IS BAD

Conflict can be good if it leads to:

- Opening up issues for discussion
- Problem-solving
- Increased involvement of team members in finding solutions
- Open, honest communication
- Release of pent-up emotions that had been passively expressed
- An increase in team spirit
- Individual growth

Unfortunately, unresolved conflict causes energy that would otherwise be devoted to work to be diverted away from it and leads to goals not being met, decreased morale, decreased cooperation among peers, intensified values difference, and irresponsible behavior.

## DEALING WITH CONFLICT

The ways in which human beings deal with conflict evolved over millions of years. Yet, how we dealt with conflict when we lived in caves does not transfer well to our modern world or to the healthcare arena! The three types of behavior humans naturally display when dealing with conflict are frequently noted in the nursing workplace. Fight or flight is a physiological reaction that occurs when a person feels that they are being threatened or attacked:

1. **Aggressive (fight):** The person attempts to keep himself or herself safe by defeating the person with whom they are in conflict. They cause disunity on the clinical unit by encouraging team members to take sides. This person talks to other team members behind another person's back. This person may yell, threaten, and attempt to ruin another nurse's reputation in either a social or professional context.
2. **Passive (flight):** The person keeps to themselves and attempts to keep safe by avoiding the conflict. Methods of communication include texting and e-mailing rather than in-person interaction. This person does not return messages and purposefully withholds information (which may cause a patient safety issue). This person does not support or help fellow staff.
3. **Unintentional (a nonstrategy):** This person internalizes the conflict and, as a result, may develop psychosomatic or anxiety-related illnesses, or manifest responses such as nervousness and crying.

The aggressive response to conflict is the most common form seen in nursing. None of these forms of behavior is effective because nurses have to work with, trust, cooperate, and communicate with fellow team members in order to provide safe, quality care. This cannot be accomplished if they are "fighting" or "flying." Nurses, in general, struggle to deal with workplace conflict. They tend to avoid dealing with issues in an open manner. Instead, they may hold onto emotions that the conflict creates (e.g., anger), but act out against others in a covert manner.

Nurses need to learn how to deal with conflict to:

■ Provide safe, high-quality patient care
■ Provide excellent customer service
■ Maintain staffing levels that would be compromised if nurses stayed away from the unit because of conflict
■ Make good decisions about patient care
■ Function in higher-level management and education settings
■ Function in a changing healthcare environment with increased stressors

Resolving conflict in a healthy manner leads to positive outcomes for the individual, team, facility, and patients. It also leads to growth and more effective problem-solving. Avoiding conflict leads to poor patient outcomes as well as ineffectual and unproductive work outcomes.

## WHAT CAUSES CONFLICT

There are three stages in the evolution of a conflict:

1. A difference in expectations arises.
2. If the difference is not resolved, it leads to discord.
3. If the discord is not resolved, it leads to dispute.

Conflict among nursing staff is often caused by:

- **Unclear roles and responsibilities:** A team member may not understand their role in the care of the patient or how to complete a task. This person doesn't understand their responsibility and attempts to figure it out on their own. To avoid this kind of misunderstanding, nurses must be clear when assigning tasks or asking for help from other team members.
- **Assumptions and expectations:** A team member may make assumptions about their role and responsibilities based on past experiences and their expectations of what is required. This person may be attempting to complete a task based on how it was completed at an earlier time and on instructions given either by a manager or by another team member. Ask open-ended questions to ascertain whether a team member is completing an assigned task based on their past experiences or whether the person is acting in response to a patient care issue of which you are unaware.
- **Differences in the core values of team members:** Disagreements among team members rarely occur because of a surface issue. Usually they are about deeper issues, such as what the team member deems as valuable. To determine what is most important to a team member, ask what they value (e.g., safe patient care, a quality job, etc.). Use the insight gained to help the person develop a solution to the issue.
- **Differences in how team members view and interpret the world around them:** Team members differ in how they view the world

and how they filter information and respond to their environment. Few people see things and respond to them in exactly the same way. By gaining insight into team members' perspectives you will better understand how they approach different problems.

- **Emotions that get in the way of conversation and effective communication:** When team members are arguing or in the midst of a conflict they are unable to reason as they normally would. Attempt to end the immediate situation, allow team members to calm down, and then approach them. Question what led to the reaction.

- **Gossiping and cliques on the unit or in the facility:** Cliques form on units and in the facility for a number of reasons. Because they have the potential to create negative repercussions for the remaining staff, the formation of cliques should be discouraged. Team members should work well together and welcome new staff. At no time should a team member be made to feel like an outsider or that they have nothing to contribute.

- **Ineffective communication:** At all times, team members should say what they mean and mean what they say. They should avoid using vague language such as "do it when you get to it" or "do whatever you think is best." This leaves the question of how to complete the task to the fellow team member's imagination, which can lead to patient safety and quality care issues as well as conflict.

- **Insufficient experience or education level of the unit manager or charge nurse:** More often than not, the unit manager or charge nurse of a particular unit has that responsibility because they were "next in line," no one else wanted the position, or the person possessed the best clinical skills among the staff. Although this person has been given a position of authority, they may not deal well with conflict or bullying (or may be the instigator of the conflict or the bully) because of limited experience or education. This person might also feel that conflict and bullying are to be expected or tolerated in nursing.

Although we may be genetically or biologically predestined to engage in or respond to conflict in a particular way, this does not mean that we must do so for the remainder of our careers. Dealing with conflict, like other topics discussed in this text, is a distinct skill that involves conscious effort to be learned.

## PRECEPTOR–PRECEPTEE CONFLICT

A preceptor may experience conflict with the preceptee for several reasons. Instances of situations that can lead to preceptor–preceptee conflict include:

- An expert in the field of nursing working with a novice in the field
- A preceptee who is unable to communicate effectively with the preceptor, leading to stress and conflict
- A preceptor who may not communicate effectively with the preceptee, leading to stress and conflict
- Dealing with a stressful work environment
- Working together closely over an extended period while dealing with personal and professional issues (both parties)
- A preceptee beginning to act independently before the preceptor is comfortable with the situation

The preceptor must be able to resolve conflict occurring in the preceptor–preceptee relationship. If conflict is not resolved, learning will be affected because of a loss of communication and trust. Conflicts that occur with one preceptee can reach into future relationships with fellow staff, future preceptees, unit managers, nursing school faculty, and others. In addition:

- If the preceptee has a bad preceptorship experience, it could lead them to feel disappointed and cynical about the profession as a whole.
- The preceptee's ability to learn will be affected because of a loss of communication and trust.
- Preceptors who experience conflict with preceptees may refuse to precept new nurses or students in the future.

If a preceptor experiences conflict with a preceptee, steps should be taken to identify the causes of the conflict and to resolve them. The following guidelines can help in preventing or dealing with conflicts in the preceptor–preceptee relationship:

- Be aware from the beginning of the preceptorship that conflict could occur. Be proactive and work to decrease and eliminate the causes.
- If conflict occurs, work immediately with the preceptee to find and eliminate the cause. Notify staff development or nursing faculty. Work together to list possible solutions for the stated

causes of the conflict. Select the best solution and work on actions to implement the solution.

■ If the preceptor cannot resolve the conflict (working with staff development and faculty as necessary), the considerations of the preceptee should take priority to salvage either a clinical rotation or new employee experience.

■ The preceptee should not be made to fear that conflict will lead to retribution from faculty, the preceptor, or staff.

# BULLYING IN NURSING

Bullying is a form of psychological violence. Although it is not physical, it is considered to be abuse and it can cause emotional harm. The term *incivility* is sometimes used in place of *bullying*; however, the two should not be confused. Incivility refers to workplace behavior that is rude or undignified. According to the Workplace Bullying Institute (WBI), it causes 12% of those surveyed to leave their jobs, whereas bullying causes 66% of those surveyed to leave theirs. Bullying occurs in all professions; unfortunately, in the healthcare industry, patients are often affected as an indirect result.

## Causes of Bullying in Nursing

■ Unsympathetic leadership; a "this is the way it has always been" mentality

■ Being a new employee (or new graduate); these individuals are at higher risk of being bullied during their first year of employment

■ A need for power and promotion

■ Lack of support from management

■ Racism, including against foreign-trained nurses

■ Support of the practice by those in authority; bullies may be protected by an informal "alliance" consisting of upper-level managers who then block any form of correction or punishment of the abusive personnel.

## Effects of Nurse Bullying on Patients

Patients may be affected indirectly by bullying in several ways:

■ Low morale and job dissatisfaction can lead to increased sick days and "mental health" days among nurses, resulting in decreased staffing and a financial burden on the institution.

- Physical symptoms caused by psychological stress affect nurses' ability to perform to the best of their ability and to provide high-quality care.
- Lack of cooperation and trust among the healthcare team leads to more errors and decreased patient safety.

## Targets of Bullying

Many of us have a picture in our mind of those who are targeted by bullies; we usually envision the target as a weak person without friends or one who did "something" to instigate the poor treatment. Quite the opposite is true. The targets of bullying are often the most skilled and independent nurses who refuse to be submissive. In healthcare facilities, they are the "gung-ho" nurses, the ones the facility and unit manager depend on to develop and complete projects. They are well-liked, skillful, honest, ethical, and are appreciated by their friends and work colleagues for being compassionate, resourceful, intelligent, warm, and empathetic. According to the WBI, "the most exploited targets are people with personalities founded on a pro-social orientation—a desire to help, heal, teach, develop, nurture others . . . they do not respond to aggressing with aggression" (WBI, 2014), and this unfortunately, is also what contributes to them being the target of a bully.

**Fast Facts**

No nurse should tolerate being the victim of a bully.

## HOW TO DEAL WITH BULLYING

The preceptor must at all times provide guidance and support and be a model of professional nursing behavior. The preceptor must be aware of facility policies dealing with unprofessional conduct and know whom to contact should their preceptee become a victim of workplace bullying. Also, the preceptee:

- Should not blame themselves for the behavior and actions of the bully. They should remember bullies choose targets they find threatening, and a threat can be anything from how the preceptee looks to a perceived threat to job security.

■ Should be encouraged to objectively document the occurrence of bullying, including what, when, where, and how. Document conversations that took place, including word-for-word quotes.

■ Should not confuse the verbal abuse that the bully uses with "constructive criticism." The preceptee should instead focus on their accomplishments and maintain self-confidence.

■ Should not respond in kind to the bully (through rude or belittling behavior), but rather continue to work to the best of their ability.

■ Should be aware of the chain of command on the unit and within the facility when reporting bullying. The preceptee should be encouraged to report the incivility immediately to a unit manager and should be aware of who to report to if the unit manager does not act or if the unit manager is the bully.

■ Should be aware of all facility policies regarding workplace professional behavior and conduct.

■ Should seek out support from a mentor or trusted friend. The preceptee can also research how to deal with a bully at www .bullyinstitute.org.

As a mentor, be open to complaints of intimidation, humiliation, belittlement, or social isolation voiced to you by the preceptee. Assure the preceptee the complaint will be handled without fear of reprisal. The preceptee should be free to verbalize issues that ultimately affect patient care. Assure them that you will work to find solutions and will bring the complaint to a higher authority if necessary. Other actions to take include:

■ If the facility does not have or does not actually follow a "zero-tolerance policy" when it comes to bullying, work to change that.

■ Encourage a "clique-less" unit. As previously noted, cliques can have a negative impact on staff retention (especially as this relates to newly employed nurses).

■ Support the target of bullying in their efforts to stand up to the abuse. Many victims of bullying do not wish to openly confront a bully because they are uncomfortable with confrontation or afraid of retaliation. Counsel the preceptee they may respond in a professional manner by making clear to the bully their wish that the behavior stop. It is important to identify the specific behavior. The victim should not state how the behavior made them feel, but instead should simply state that they wish the behavior to stop and that if it continues it will be reported to a superior. However, no confrontation should take place without the nurse manager, faculty member, and/or preceptor being present.

- Encourage the new nurse to report episodes of bullying to human resources or, in the case of the nursing student, per school policy, as appropriate.
- Allow the process of reporting to occur, including the process for superiors to deal with the unprofessional behavior, and support the preceptee during the process.
- Suggest counseling for the victim if they express a need for it because of emotional trauma that may have been endured.

## References

Hiemer, A. (2011). Conflict resolution. *RN Journal*. Retrieved from https://rn-journal.com/journal-of-nursing/conflict-resolution

Workplace Bullying Institute. (2014). Retrieved from https://workplace bullying.org/

## Bibliography

Ciocco, M. (2018). *Fast facts on nurse bullying, incivility and workplace violence*. New York, NY: Springer Publishing Company.

# 14

# Helping the Preceptee Deal With Reality Shock

*Remember how it was to begin your first job as a nurse? As a new nurse, you were eager to be on your own, to meet your fellow staff and begin to make new friends, to begin the career you worked so hard to achieve and to finally be a "real nurse." During preceptorship, the new nurse is guided and somewhat protected by the preceptor. Although the new nurse may experience disappointment during preceptorship, "shock" usually does not set in until some months after preceptorship has finished and the nurse is on their own. The preceptor can prepare new nurses for the onset of "reality shock" and help them work through the phases they will encounter.*

After reading this chapter, the reader will be able to:

1. Define *reality shock*
2. Describe the causes of reality shock
3. List the stages of reality shock
4. List three activities to assist the new nurse in the shock phase
5. List three activities to assist the new nurse in the recovery phase

## REALITY SHOCK DEFINED

According to Businessdictionary.com, reality shock is the "unsettling or jarring experience resulting from wide disparity between what was expected and what the real situation turns out to be, such as the first day on a new job." Understand it is a normal process experienced by new graduates of all professions when they first begin work.

In nursing, reality shock starts several months into the job, usually around the 3- to 6-month mark. Some nursing journals and entries in online blogs hold that reality shock is just the shock of reality, or of working in the real world. It is true that there is a feeling of shock when transitioning from school to work. However, the shock is worse in some facilities where the new nurse is dealing with bullying as well as verbal, physical, and mental abuse and witnessing inadequate and unsafe care of patients. Reality shock and accompanying stresses can lead new nurses to doubt their chosen profession and their abilities. If these feelings continue, the new nurse can leave the profession. Understanding which phase of reality shock the preceptee is experiencing will help to plan interventions and teaching strategies. These should change when the phase changes.

## CAUSES OF REALITY SHOCK FOR NURSES

Since Marlene Kramer's book *Reality Shock: Why Nurses Leave Nursing* was published in 1974, the causes of reality shock have not changed. In fact, they have only multiplied. The turnover rate in nursing within the first year of employment remains high. Because of this and possibly due to Kramer's study, many hospitals developed programs such as nurse internships, clearly-prescribed preceptorship programs, residency programs, awards and recognition for facility and individual nursing practice, and continuing education.

Still, new nurses face a variety of issues that lead to reality shock. These issues are similar to or worse than those faced by nurses over 40 years ago, and it is disappointing to think very little progress has been made despite new programs. Contributors to reality shock include:

- Feeling that the "real world" of working in healthcare is not similar to what one was taught in nursing school

- Feeling as though one was not thoroughly prepared to care for patients, or has not been given "real-world" scenarios in training
- High nurse-to-patient ratios
- High patient acuity
- Shortened or nonexistent orientation periods, especially in long-term care and subacute areas
- Too much to do on a given shift, with repercussions for overtime
- Not being able to spend time with patients
- Mistreatment—verbal, physical, or both—by fellow staff, administration, and physicians
- Bullying

## PHASES OF REALITY SHOCK AND HOW TO TRANSITION THROUGH THEM

The new nurse will pass through four phases of reality shock: honeymoon, shock, recovery, and resolution. One of your responsibilities as preceptor and mentor is to help the preceptee understand they will experience reality shock. Explain what reality shock is, how the preceptee can prepare, and how they can respond. Another responsibility of the preceptor is to assist new nurses through each stage by helping them to develop coping mechanisms and to make them aware of available resources. Although preceptorship may long be over when the new nurse experiences reality shock, you can help the preceptee recognize when it occurs, what it is, and how to cope. Some suggestions keyed to each phase follow.

### Honeymoon Phase

In this initial phase, preceptees are happy to be starting their new job. They are happy to meet fellow staff members and view all members of the team as dynamic professionals as eager to work as they are. They are enthusiastic to learn and care for patients, and state they are very happy with both their profession and clinical area. They are highly focused on learning new skills, developing their roles, and meeting new members of the healthcare team.

### *How to Help*

- Recognize they may be overconfident and help them remain grounded. Review the "rules" of preceptorship, emphasizing they may not perform care not observed by you first.

- Encourage the preceptee to bond with you as their preceptor/ mentor, but also introduce them to other registered nurses (RNs) who may serve as mentors.
- Introduce the preceptee to other members of the staff with similar backgrounds and interests to encourage beginning friendships.
- Celebrate the successes and goals attained by the preceptee.
- Enjoy the enthusiasm the preceptee has for the job and the work they are doing, and channel this energy into learning new skills. Don't stifle their enthusiasm, but remain realistic.
- Remember the three-goal rule so that they are learning new experiences gradually and realistically.
- Let them know that there is a difference between what they need to know now and what can be learned later so that they are not overwhelmed by what all there is to know!
- Interject realism into daily work and keep the preceptee focused on patient care routines.

## Shock Phase

Preceptees begin to see the flaws within the healthcare system and the facility. They notice fellow healthcare workers take shortcuts of which they disapprove. They see fellow staff as disorganized, lazy, and inattentive and may become concerned about the practices of other nurses. This phase can begin during preceptorship and may be brought about after they witness something upsetting for the learner such as a patient care incident, an error that they commit, or receiving negative feedback from another nurse. Other concerns include:

- Discovering that the preceptor does not know everything; possibly witnessing the preceptor taking shortcuts in care that were not taught in nursing school, or not following policies and procedures that they had emphasized that the preceptee follow
- Discovering at times they do not have the tools and supplies necessary to care for patients according to the methods they were taught in nursing school
- Discovering communication issues that may develop among staff
- Encountering fellow nurses who do not act in a professional manner
- Experiencing being mentally "hurt," harassed, embarrassed, or bullied by a health team member
- Experiencing a situation that leads them to feel angry, disillusioned, or humiliated

- They now have low energy or enthusiasm and lack motivation and self-confidence. They become discouraged.
- Their anxiety level increases.
- They may become disorganized.
- They question themselves and their chosen profession.

### How to Help

- Be aware that this phase follows the honeymoon phase and that the preceptee may experience (and verbalize) unhappiness and frustration with the new job and fellow staff.
- Avoid teaching new or complex skills. Because of anxiety, learning may be difficult.
- Don't assign highly acute or complex patient care to them.
- Avoid time pressures on their patient care.
- Remind them that all nurses go through this phase. Share stories of your own experiences and that the preceptee will make it through.
- Emphasize their successes and relate how far they have come and how well they are doing.
- Realize that they may be going through this phase without showing the signs of it. They have internalized their fears.
- Let them know that they will find their niche in nursing.
- Listen as the preceptee verbalizes what they have found troubling.
- Continue to model professional behavior; do not take shortcuts in care or encourage others to do so.
- Assist the preceptee in finding supplies and equipment when needed. If an item is not available, channel the frustration that the preceptee may be experiencing into approaching the administration with ideas and suggestions for new or additional equipment.
- Allow the preceptee to verbalize and vent frustrations, but in a constructive manner, not a "bitch session." The goal of such interactions should be that the preceptee can vent but must also develop a solution to the problem and a plan for how to enact it.

### Recovery Phase

Preceptees realize there are both positive and negative aspects of the profession, some of which they can work on to improve. They should also realize there are some things they will not be able to change but must adapt to. They establish realistic expectations for their fellow staff and realize not all nurses will act in a professional manner or follow facility standards for care. They realize that what is important is that they themselves act professionally and provide safe, quality care for their patients. The new nurse begins to define what type of nurse they want to be and realizes that they must remain true to these goals and expectations. They are now able to better manage their care and skills. New skills are developing and they require less supervision.

### How to Help

- Always treat the preceptee with kindness and respect.
- Help the preceptee deal with situations realistically.
- Suggest the preceptee document the improvements they would like to see take place and assist in working through the development and proposals steps.
- Insist the preceptee not be removed from preceptorship and given their own assignment until the preceptorship is completed. The frustration and fear felt at being given an assignment too early could lead the preceptee to leave the position.
- Continue to act as the preceptee's advocate.
- Do not degrade or speak unkindly about fellow staff in front of the preceptee. Encourage the preceptee to always treat fellow healthcare team members with respect.
- Continue to utilize critical thinking exercises.
- Continue to remind them of how far they have come.
- Provide more detailed feedback as they should now be ready to hear and manage more information as their anxiety levels are decreasing.
- Continue to set new goals, continuing the three new goal rule.
- Use your sense of humor to help preceptees regain theirs.

### Resolution

At this stage, preceptees may feel it is easier to "give in" and adopt the poor or unsafe work ethic they find in their fellow staff to "fit in." The preceptor/mentor must step in and help the preceptee retain their values and goals. Help the preceptee to understand there is a balance between nursing school and the "real world," and they should not be willing to compromise patient safety or quality of care. They should begin to feel they "fit in" with the unit staff. This stage may not occur until after preceptorship has ended and they have experienced 1 to 2 years of professional practice.

### How to Help

- Help the preceptee identify and manage conflicts (see Chapter 12, The Unsafe Preceptee and How to Avoid "Failure to Fail").
- Assist the preceptee with problem-solving.
- Point out what is working well and continue to celebrate successes and goals attained.
- Help the preceptee to identify resources that can be of assistance as they resolve conflicts and works through issues.
- Instruct them on how to create change in nursing practice on the unit or facility.
- Assure them that if they are not satisfied with their current work experience, they can change as their career progresses and find their "niche" in nursing.

### Fast Facts

Still of significance is Patricia Benner's book, *From Novice to Expert.* Written in 1984, the work is based on the findings of Marlene Kramer. It is mandatory reading for all nurse educators and preceptors.

### How to Help Throughout All Phases

The following suggestions will help the preceptee throughout all phases of preceptorship. Review the basics:

- Encourage the preceptee to become as familiar with the unit as possible during orientation/preceptorship. This means schedules, location of supplies, fellow team members, and so on.
- Reassure the preceptee reality shock is a normal process experienced by all nurses in varying degrees.
- If your facility uses only one shift for preceptorship, suggest the following change: Split the preceptorship between the day shift (7 a.m. to 3 p.m., or 7 a.m. to 7 p.m.); then, after initial goals have been achieved and the preceptee can confidently care for a typical assignment of patients, switch the preceptee to the

shift for which they were hired (the preceptee should change preceptors at this point). Several learning goals will be achieved. The preceptee:

- Will understand the workings of the previous shift
- Will have staff development resources available at the beginning of the preceptorship, when they are becoming familiar with the unit and facility
- Will become familiar (while still on preceptorship) with the shift during which they will work, thus increasing the preceptee's comfort level
- Will become familiar with the staff with whom they will be working, including assistive personnel, before the end of preceptorship

- As stated in Chapter 5, Critical Thinking Skills, ensure that the preceptee knows the location of all policy and procedure, Safety Data Sheet (SDS), intravenous, pharmacy, and emergency manuals. Review the contents of each before the end of preceptorship.
- Review how to contact all facility resources.
- Review the protocol for reporting medication errors or equipment malfunction.
- Review the information covered in Chapter 6, Organizing the Clinical Day, and ensure the preceptee is comfortable phoning physicians and other healthcare team members before having the preceptee do this on their own.
- Assure the new nurse you will remain their mentor, even after preceptorship is over. Encourage the preceptee to reach out to you if they need assistance or have questions.
- Arrange for the preceptee to meet the new shift preceptor (if this type of preceptorship is offered at your facility) before moving to the new shift. Be available to the preceptee for questions and issues after preceptorship is over.
- Introduce the preceptee to fellow RNs who can serve as role models. Review the section in Chapter 1, Preceptorship in a Nutshell, that speaks to the qualities of a mentor.
- Prior to the end of preceptorship, review all state, facility, and unit guidelines regarding the RN scope of practice. Reiterate with the preceptee they must adhere to these guidelines at all times. The RN is ultimately responsible for following all guidelines and can be held accountable if they are not followed

- If the preceptee is still a student, encourage them to seek out nurse internship opportunities in the facility where they wish to work. This will assist the preceptee in the transition.
- Be aware of signs the preceptee is moving through the different phases of reality shock, and especially those indicating that they are reaching the shock phase.
- As reviewed in Chapter 7, Prioritization and Communication, continue to provide feedback.
- Many new nurses feel similar frustrations and fears when beginning their first job. Acknowledge that the preceptee may be feeling the following, and encourage ongoing communication:
  - Lack of confidence when performing skills and taking care of patients
  - Struggling to acquire critical thinking skills
  - Developing relationships with peers and preceptors
  - Attempting to be independent immediately, but lacking skills and knowledge to do so
  - Frustrations with the work environment (unit, facility, organization), including lack of supplies, lack of continuing education, perceived lack of opportunity to advance, lack of support
  - Organization and priority setting
  - Communicating with physicians and other members of the healthcare team
- The preceptor should share stories of how they felt when beginning the first job and how they coped. Included should be issues and situations that were faced, and how the preceptor resolved problems, dealt with unprofessional behavior of staff, learned from mistakes, and passed through the phases of reality shock.

## Fast Facts

Kramer suggests that during the shock phase, nurses should ask themselves two questions: (a) What must I do to become the nurse I really want to be? (b) What must I do so that my nursing contributes to my patients and the community? Answering these questions will assist nurses in establishing priorities and keeping them on the course to becoming the nurse that they envisioned.

**Fast Facts**

Throughout preceptorship and when speaking to fellow staff, make a conscious choice to present a realistic, honest view of the unit, facility, and organization where you all work. Do not speak in derogatory tones, but rather emphasize where improvement can be made and how all can work together to make it happen.

### References

Benner, P. (1984). *From novice to expert: Excellence and power in clinical nursing practice.* Menlo Park, CA: Addison-Wesley.

Kramer, M. (1974). *Reality shock: Why nurses leave nursing.* St. Louis, MO: Mosby.

# 15

# Preparing for the Future

*The preceptor can assist the preceptee in preparing for future employment or advancing their career. For example, the preceptor can explain the importance of and assist with portfolio development, as well as making the preceptee aware of continuing education opportunities available within the facility and within the practice specialty. If the nurse is a diploma or associate degree graduate, the preceptor can explain the importance of attaining a BSN degree and beyond. At all times, the preceptor should promote continuing education and professional involvement. It is also important to promote certification in your specialty and introduce other members of the nursing team who are certified.*

After reading this chapter, the reader will be able to:

1. List the types of portfolios
2. List 10 items to include in a professional portfolio
3. Describe a growth and development portfolio
4. Describe the importance of certification
5. Describe the importance of attaining a BSN and beyond

## RÉSUMÉ VERSUS CURRICULUM VITAE (CV): WHAT IS THE DIFFERENCE?

Both résumés and CVs are used when applying for jobs or to showcase achievements. They are, however, not interchangeable. A CV is usually longer and there is no limit as to how many pages it may contain. It is more in depth in its detailing of accomplishments, education, professional affiliation, job history, publications, professional projects, honors, and awards. All aspects of the CV are listed chronologically, with the most recent accomplishment first, in sections with separate headings. The CV does not change to adapt to a different position; rather, the cover letter to the CV should be adapted to the position to which the applicant is applying.

A résumé is shorter than the CV—usually one page. It should not document an entire job history, but rather briefly describe a person's skills and job experience. The résumé should be changed to adapt to the position to which the applicant is applying.

CVs and résumés serve different purposes in different parts of the world. For example, a CV is used when applying for an academic position, but it is also used in place of a résumé in parts of Europe. The preceptee should also be prepared to submit a résumé to some graduate schools as part of the application process.

## PORTFOLIO DEVELOPMENT

In years past, nursing portfolios were completed as a school project at the BSN or MSN level. The concept was simple: collect all the documentation requested and place it along with a résumé or CV in a large plastic file box within neatly labeled folders. Nurses were then graded on the content and organization of the portfolio. Although portfolios were traditionally completed by various other professionals, such as artists, architects, and models, the nursing field really didn't grasp the concept of portfolio development and its value to the profession until fairly recently. Portfolios have now become part of the capstone project of many schools and are formatted to "follow" the student from graduation to job application.

There are several different types of portfolios, but only two main formats. Both are outlined in this chapter.

## Professional Portfolio

Portfolio development and maintenance is an important aspect of the professional growth of the nurse. Although a résumé or CV provides basic information about a nurse's career and education, the portfolio backs up and supports the résumé, CV, or information expressed in a verbal interview. The preceptor can assist the new nurse in the development of their professional portfolio. Professional portfolios:

- Contain documents that prove a nurse's competence and expertise
- Are used for promotions, job applications (they are now an expected part of the job application process), licensure/relicensure, school applications, performance reviews, certification application and renewal, clinical ladder advancement, accreditation survey needs, and continuing education
- Are meant to be seen and reviewed by others (necessitating an organized, clear, concise format)
- Should include copies of documents such as contact hour certificates and facility- or unit-specific competencies; keeping these documents in the portfolio helps ensure they aren't lost or omitted when there is a change in jobs
- Can be designed and redesigned to demonstrate, highlight, and address specific aspects of one's career as it evolves, and should be updated periodically, depending on the goals of the nurse
- Should include documents and projects that demonstrate problem-solving and critical thinking skills as well as competence in a specialty

## Growth and Development Portfolio

A growth and development portfolio aids the nurse in their self-development process. This type of portfolio:

- Contains collected documents and materials that provide evidence of professional development
- Is used to house information that will eventually be placed in the professional portfolio
- Acts as a guide for the nurse to monitor what has been completed and what goals and competencies still need to be met
- Can contain logs that the nurse designs that may list education programs they have completed and tracking required for contact hours for licensure and certification
- Is meant to only be seen by the nurse and not shared with others

## Steps in Portfolio Development

Oermann (2002) likened the development of a portfolio to the nursing process, with the nurse moving through four steps: assessment, planning, implementation, and evaluation. The preceptor can assist nurses in moving through this process. They can make them aware of educational opportunities that exist at their institution and in their specialty area, professional affiliations, or associations that it would be beneficial to obtain or join, accreditation goals for the nurse and the facility, and competency development. These actions are in keeping with Robert Wood Johnson Foundation (RWJF)/Institute of Medicine (The National Academies of Science, Engineering and Medicine "The National Academies" formerly the IOM) recommendations that nurses engage in lifelong learning. The portfolio development process includes:

- **Assessment:** Assess the preceptee's learning needs to ascertain what areas require further development; identify specific goals to be met.
- **Planning:** Assist the preceptee in developing a plan to meet learning needs. The preceptor can assist by making the preceptee aware of in-service and continuing education opportunities available in the facility, within the specialty area, and in the state nursing organization. Introduce the preceptee to the members of the nursing education department, specifically to the nurse educator within your specialty area. Nurse educators should also take an interest in advancing the preceptee and in helping them to achieve short-term and long-term learning goals. Be sure to make the preceptee aware of the various other types of learning opportunities, such as specialty-relevant articles or a new skill to achieve.
- **Implementation:** After the preceptee has assessed their learning needs and formulated goals, they should implement the plan (i.e., complete the activities they have planned). Help the preceptee develop goals and assist in establishing completion dates for activities. Encourage the preceptee to gather the documentation that provides evidence of the educational activities they have completed.
- **Evaluation:** The last step of the process is evaluation. Did the preceptee meet their goals or do they need to revise the overall

plan? All documentation can be reviewed to ascertain if the learning need was met or if more development needs to take place. The plan that was initially developed should have accompanying documentation proving that the goal was met.

## Fast Facts

The preceptor should build time into the orientation schedule to allow the preceptee to participate in educational events. New nurses (actually, all nurses) become frustrated when they have planned to attend an educational event within their facility and are unable to participate because of staffing or other constraints.

## What Should Be Placed in a Portfolio?

The portfolio should represent the nurse and their professional and academic accomplishments. It should include:

- A document containing contact information and license number and a brief biography
- A professionally prepared and updated CV or résumé; this document should also be maintained and updated electronically.
- A list of professional and personal references with their titles and contact information
- At least three to four letters of reference on professional letterhead. Letters should be unique and signed and not copies of one letter with different signatures. References can be from current and former employers, current or former faculty, preceptors, mentors, and professional colleagues.
- A document outlining professional goals and objectives
- Unofficial copies of school transcripts
- Copies of nursing licenses
- A list of the professional organizations to which the nurse belongs, with roles in national, state, or local nursing organizations noted (i.e., member, officer, or committee member); and offices or committee memberships held in the past. If the portfolio is being developed by a student nurse, it should also include activities

within student nurse national, state, and facility organizations, and membership in any honor societies.

- For all continuing education credits and certifications attained, note the reason for attendance to facilitate review of this information with the person evaluating the portfolio.
- Contact hour and continuing education certificates. Maintain a record of how many hours have been attained. As of this date, only 20 states require contact hours for re-licensure; however, other states are beginning to follow the trend.
- Seminar literature, such as an agenda or outline
- Staff development programs
- In-service training
- National certifications attained, with copies of certificates
- School courses completed (transcripts or academic evaluations)
- Copies of published articles or books written, co-written, or edited, and any written work completed for an employer, including developed and written policies, brochures, and fliers for patient and staff education, instructional manuals, and PowerPoint presentations
- Documented examples of completed projects
- Honors and awards received, including the title, organization from which received, date received, and why the award was received. What was done to be recognized or nominated for the award? Be able to verbalize this to a future employer or school representative.
- Volunteer and community service work. List the organizations and committees and work completed for the organization. Document how work for the organization enhances the role of the professional nurse.

### Fast Facts

Pursing continuing education, even if the facility or state licensing board does not require it, demonstrates a willingness to keep current in the profession.

Smith (2011) notes that portfolios should include samples of work that showcases the following:

| Quality | Example |
| --- | --- |
| Critical thinking skills | A care plan developed for a unique type of patient with rationales and interventions |
| Problem-solving skills, communication style | Team conferences |
| Leadership | Evaluations written, staffing assignments with rationale |
| Team and group work | Working as a team member on a difficult project, efforts in collaboration |
| Time management | Rationalize care priorities in patient care or professional work |
| Caring | Copies of thank you notes, student evaluations |
| Clinical skills | A list of clinical skills completed, including lab sign-off sheets, competencies attained, and preceptor courses or projects |

For clinical skills, note practicum and preceptorship programs completed. Include the location, contact information for the preceptor, letters of reference from the preceptor, and or areas/units worked. Be able to verbally address the goals of the program and skills achieved.

## The Electronic Portfolio

Many universities are offering their students, faculty, and alumni the opportunity to develop an e-portfolio (electronic or digital portfolio). This type of portfolio is completed using dedicated software or web-based programs, either for free or for payment to an outside service. These programs assist in the collection and organization of documents. Preparation of an e-portfolio is now considered part of the scholarly process in many fields, including nursing. The concept of document and project (sometimes called "artifact") collection and showcasing is the same as in traditional portfolio preparation; however, the e-portfolio offers many advantages over a paper portfolio. For example, an e-portfolio:

- Is cloud-based, so it will not deteriorate or be destroyed
- Can be updated within minutes
- Can be reproduced easily and clearly

- Provides a dynamic, not static, representation of skills, competencies, and achievements
- Can be searched and accessed easily by multiple parties
- Enables more than one party to access and upload information (e.g., groups working together on a project)
- Easily changes layouts depending on goals (e.g., to showcase competencies to a potential employer, to showcase projects to an accrediting body)
- Includes an area for reflective blog development

**Fast Facts**

A preceptor portfolio is unique to the role of a preceptor. It should include examples of education achieved, teaching experiences, and preceptorship involvement. Selected items should prove professional and personal growth as a preceptor (Clark, 2019; Willis, 2017).

## CERTIFICATION

There are over 200 nursing specialties and subspecialties, many of which have certifying bodies. By definition, certification is the formal process by which a certifying body such as the American Nurses Credentialing Center (ANCC) or American Association of Critical-Care Nurses (AACN) "validates a nurse's knowledge, skills, and abilities in a defined role and clinical area of practice, based on predetermined standards. Nurses achieve certification credentials through specialized education, experience in a specialty area, and a qualifying exam" (ANCC, 2010). Certification sets the nurse apart from their peers. It recognizes the nurse has gained expertise and denotes the pursuit of excellence through continuing education and skill development. Assist the preceptee in researching how to achieve certification in their particular area of interest. Encourage the preceptee to attain and maintain certification.

Benefits of certification include:

- Recognition by peers, supervisors, and administration in the healthcare field for competence and excellence in practice

- Professional achievement
- Continuing education
- Career advancement (ladder progression, job promotion, and increased "hire-ability")
- Networking opportunities
- Professional contribution that benefits patients and fellow professionals
- Personal accomplishment
- Competitive edge in the job market
- Increased salary and job opportunities
- Potential for increased patient satisfaction and decreased patient care errors
- Demonstration of commitment and professional growth

## THE IMPORTANCE OF A BACHELOR'S DEGREE AND BEYOND

The National Academies of Science, Engineering and Medicine (The National Academies) recommends nurses should "achieve higher levels of education and training in order to respond to the demands of an evolving health care system and to meet the changing needs of patients" (IOM & RWJF, 2011). It recommends increasing the proportion of nurses with a baccalaureate degree based on the following criteria:

- Healthcare delivery in the United States is changing.
- The traditional role of the registered nurse (RN) as the bedside caregiver and the hospital as the accepted site for healthcare delivery will no longer be the norm.
- Healthcare delivery is moving to outpatient and community settings, which will require a greater number of clinical specialists.
- There is a greater need for nurse practitioners and other advanced generalists to provide healthcare that is more accessible and affordable to the public and especially the underserved.
- There is a greater need for nurse educators and researchers and those nurses holding doctoral degrees.

It is not enough for nursing schools or colleges to simply increase their enrollments and graduate larger numbers of basically prepared nurses. There is an increased need for nurses with expertise in health promotion, disease prevention, case management, and managed care to work not only in hospitals and subacute settings but also in what had been considered nontraditional settings, such as health maintenance organizations (HMOs), community and outpatient centers, schools, nursing school-operated clinics, the workplace, and the home. In tandem with these changes:

- Nurses are to function more independently in decision-making and case management as well as still performing their traditional roles.
- Nurses must be able to communicate effectively with all members of the healthcare team, patients, and their families, but be competent in the roles of provider, designer, manager, and coordinator of care (American Association of Colleges of Nursing [AACN], 2014).
- The skill sets the RN requires include being able to delegate care as well as planning and integrating treatment for patients across multiple settings.

In this context, the AACN concludes, "registered nurses at the entry-level of professional practice should possess, at a minimum, the educational preparation provided by a four-year Bachelor of Science degree program in nursing (BSN)" (AACN, 2014).

Students graduating from a baccalaureate degree program are prepared to practice in all healthcare settings because, unlike their colleagues from diploma or associate degree programs, they have had preparation broader in range and includes education in "clinical, scientific, decision making, and humanistic skills, including preparation in community health, patient education, and nursing management and leadership . . . these skills are essential for today's professional nurse who must make quick, sometimes life-and-death decisions; design and manage a comprehensive plan of nursing care; understand a patient's treatment, symptoms, and danger signs; supervise other nursing personnel and support staff; master advanced technology; guide patients through the maze of health care resources in a community; and educate patients on health care options and how to adopt healthy lifestyles" (AACN, 2014).

As of 2020, only New York State requires the BSN as an entry into practice and other states are proposing that a nurse attain a BSN within 10 years of initial licensure in order to meet the growing need for BSN-prepared nurses. Those nurses can then more easily move into master's and doctoral programs. Hospitals attempting to attain AACN Magnet status are also requiring their current nurses to obtain a BSN by set deadlines, and many others are not hiring new graduates unless they have graduated from a baccalaureate program or are in the process of obtaining their degree.

Baccalaureate-prepared nurses are being "utilized in ways that recognize their different educational preparation and competency from other entry-level RNs" (AACN, 2014). According to the AACN, the BSN-prepared nurse:

- Provides more complex aspects of daily care and patient education
- Designs and coordinates a comprehensive plan of nursing care for the entire length of a patient's stay
- Designs discharge and teaching plans for patients
- Collaborates with patients, physicians, family members, and other hospital departments and resource personnel

## Fast Facts

The preceptor should encourage the new nurse or student to continue with their education not only to meet the demands of a changing healthcare system, but to also continue delivering safe, high-quality, evidence-based practice care to their patients.

### Nurse Residency Programs

The preceptor who is with the senior nursing student should strongly encourage them to begin work in a facility that possesses a nurse residency program. The Bureau of Labor Statistics has predicted that for the years 2012 to 2022, there will be 525,000 nurses retiring and a need for 1.05 million new nurses by 2022 (Chant & Westendorf, 2019). Nurses may enter the workforce directly without being adequately prepared because they now must meet the staffing demands of the facility where they were hired. Although these nurses are enthusiastic about starting their new careers, they quickly burn out from the stress and at least 37% of them leave the profession by their second anniversary (Chant & Westendorf, 2019). Studies have shown that nurse residency programs may improve nurse retention and satisfaction. Nurse residency programs were also recommended by The

Institute of Medicine in 2011 as a way to support newly graduated nurses and their entry to practice.

Nurse residency programs should have:

- Facility support and "buy-in"
- Facility leadership committed to the ongoing successful operation of the program
- Resources dedicated specifically to the program including personnel specific to the program who will assist the graduate nurses and their transition into practice (i.e., program coordinator and educators)
- A healthy work environment free from bullying and incivility; one in which nursing is a valued part of the healthcare community
- Strong support of the current nursing staff
- A strong, evidence-based curriculum including skills, competency development, emphasis on patient safety, clinical leadership, professional development, and development of critical thinking skills
- A continually assessed evaluation process to ensure implementation of suggested improvements
- A healthcare team that promotes nursing professionalism and nurtures new staff nurses and students
- Access for the new nurses to attend continuing education events, take part in peer support, networking and other team and self-building activities
- Clearly defined outcomes and objectives with measurable overall goals
- Formally educated preceptors dedicated to the program and an availability of mentors, both of whom act to support, train, and socialize the new nurse
- Classroom portion that allows for new nurse interaction, support and networking with peers and review of case studies, simulation, clinical debriefing, and competency testing
- Clinical immersion that allows for the development of skill competence

### References

American Association of Colleges of Nursing. (2014). *The baccalaureate degree in nursing as minimal preparation for professional practice.* Retrieved from http://www.aacn.nche.edu/publications/position/bacc-degree-prep

American Nurses Credentialing Center. (2010). *Why certify? The benefits of nursing certification.* Retrieved from http://www.medscape.com/view article/717805

Chant, K. J., & Westendorf, D. S. (2019). Nurse residency programs: Key components for sustainability. *Journal for Nurses in Professional Development, 35*(4), 185–192. doi:10.1097/NND.0000000000000560

Clark, M. (2019, April). The importance of a professional nursing portfolio. *HealthLeaders.* Retrieved from https://www.healthleadersmedia.com /nursing/importance-professional-nursing-portfolio

Institute of Medicine & the Robert Wood Johnson Foundation. (2011). *Initiative on the future of nursing.* Retrieved from https://pubmed.ncbi .nlm.nih.gov/24983041/

Oermann, M. H. (2002). Developing a professional portfolio in nursing. *Orthopaedic Nursing, 21*(2), 73–78. Retrieved from www.nursing-informatics .com/Oermann.pdf

Smith, L. S. (2011). Showcase your talents with a career portfolio. *Nursing, 41*(7), 54–56. doi:10.1097/01.NURSE.0000398641.62631.8e

Willis, K. (2017, November 24). *How to perfect your nursing portfolio: What is it, what goes in it, and what should you do with it?* Retrieved from https:// www.paysa.com/blog/how-to-perfect-your-nursing-portfolio-what-is-it -what-goes-in-it-and-what-should-you-do-with-it/

# IV

# Problem-Solving and Clinical Tools

# 16

# Preceptorship Competency Forms and Clinical Tools

*This chapter contains the forms mentioned throughout the text.*

After reading this chapter, the reader will be able to:

1. Verbalize the rights of medication administration
2. Verbalize actions to take before and after receiving a patient care report
3. List five skills of critical thinking
4. List the steps of the SBAR system
5. List the steps of the Five-Minute Preceptor

## MEDICATION ADMINISTRATION

### The Right Patient

- Identifies the patient using the facility-approved method (may include a combination of two identifiers, such as full name and birth date, picture, or bar code system).
- Checks the patient's *full* name against the med sheets/medication administration record (MAR) and original order.
- Verifies allergies with the patient verbally and with the MAR.

## The Right Medication

- Checks the medication label against the original order.
- Checks the medication against the order at least three times: When removing the medication from the dispensing system, when pouring the medication, and prior to administering the medication.

## The Right Dose

- Checks the order and confirms that the dose is correct (uses a drug reference manual or computer application if necessary).
- If a drug calculation is necessary, asks another nurse to also calculate the dose to be sure it is correct (confirm this possible policy in your institution and review with the preceptee).

## The Right Route or the Right Form

- Checks the order against the med sheet/MAR and confirms that the route is correct.
- If the patient is unable to tolerate the medication by the ordered route, researches whether the route or type of medication can be changed.
- *Never* crushes a medication that should not be crushed.
- *Never* mixes crushed medications together to expedite the administration process (e.g., a patient with a gastrostomy tube [G-tube]).

## The Right Time

- Ensures that the ordered times correspond with facility policy. Understands that administrating a medication too late or too early constitutes a medication error.
- If giving a PRN (*pro re nata*, or as-needed) medication, confirms when the last dose was given and that the dose is being given within the appropriate time frame.
- Ensures that the medication is being administered on the correct date.

## The Right Documentation

- Does not pre-sign for a medication. Signs for a medication only *after* it is given.

- Does not wait until the end of the shift to sign for medications given or to enter the information in the electronic medical record (EMR). This will prevent inadvertent double dosing of the patient by either self or another nurse.
- When necessary, includes any other vital information having to do with the administration of a medication; for example, site given, laboratory results (international normalized ratio [INR]), or vital signs (heart rate, respirations, or blood pressure).

### The Right Reason

- Verbalizes the rationale for the medication being administered. Familiarizes themselves with the patient's history and why the medication is ordered.
- Questions the medication order if it is not compatible with the patient's history or current condition.
- Verbalizes why the medication is being given and its desired (and adverse) effects. Recognizes when they are not knowledgeable and seeks answers through drug literature or the pharmacist on staff.

### The Right Response

- After administering the medication, determines whether the desired response was achieved.
- Follows appropriate timeline for reassessment after administering PRN medications (e.g., ascertains patient's temperature after 30 to 60 minutes; pain medication after 1 hour, or as per facility guidelines).
- Documents the patient's response to the medication and other interventions. Reports if the response is not appropriate or not reached.

## INITIAL ORGANIZATION REVIEW CHECK-OFF LIST

### Before Obtaining Report

- Introduces self to patient.
- Verifies patient ID as per facility policy.
- Checks orders written in the past 24 hours and any orders or treatments that need to be carried out during the shift.

- Checks schedules for therapy and surgery.
- Checks MAR for preoperative/pretherapy medication schedule and also scheduled meds.
- Verbalizes that they will assess the patient before treatment and/or therapy for need of pain medication.
- Notes if any medications are missing from the patient medication dispensing system. If medications are missing, notifies pharmacy and does not borrow from another patient or dispensing system on another unit.
- Ascertains when PRNs were last administered and whether the patient is due for any PRN medications.
- Ascertains if treatments must be completed before the patient leaves the unit, and when any treatments are scheduled to be done during the shift.
- Briefly assesses the patient's orientation, general state, and stability and ensures that there are no immediate problems.
- Ascertains any immediate patient needs (e.g., pain medication).
- Lists needs or questions to refer to during report.

### After Obtaining Report

- Makes a list of what is to be accomplished during the shift.
- Introduces self to the patient (if not done previously).
- Provides for privacy.
- Explains care to be provided.
- Notes problems or issues immediately addressed before the shift began.
- Completes either a focused or a more thorough head-to-toe assessment. Begins with patients who may be leaving the unit for a test, therapy, or surgery or those most recently admitted.
- Assesses mental status, skin color, breathing effort, and facial symmetry while speaking to the patient.
- Checks intravenous lines, enteral feedings, Foley catheters, chest tubes, suction, drains, wound vacs, etc.
- Checks that all monitors, pumps, specialty beds, and other patient care equipment is working correctly. Verbalizes the action to take for removing nonworking equipment from service.
- Ensures that the infusing intravenous solutions are correct and infusing at the correct rate. Zeroes out the amount infused as per facility policy.
- Notes the amount left in bottle/bag (LIB) of any intravenous fluid.

- Traces lines and tubing back to the patient and assesses insertion sites, noting any signs of inflammation and infection.
- Notes the amount of suction, urinary drainage, wound drainage, etc. Notes the amount, consistency, odor, and color of any drainage.
- Performs a safety check. Places the call light in reach and the, bed in the lowest position, with side rails up or as per unit/facility policy.
- Places patient belongings and necessary items within easy reach of the patient (e.g., glasses, tissues, phone, and water).

### After Checking All Patients

- Communicates abnormal assessment findings appropriately.
- Documents initial patient findings.
- Begins to prioritize activities to be completed during the shift.

## CRITICAL THINKING EVALUATION CHECK-OFF LIST

Adopted from Alfaro-Lefevre (2008), Rubenfeld and Scheffer (2015), and Banning (2006), the following are examples of critical thinking behaviors. Answering "yes" to a point indicates that the preceptee is employing skills of critical thinking. If not, encourage the preceptee to do so.

### Is the Preceptee

- Curious and inquisitive? Asking questions and seeking answers in order to learn more?
- Communicating effectively (all forms of communication)?
- Open-minded and fair in dealings with other members of the healthcare team?
- Able to distinguish what is an accurate or inaccurate inference?
- Using analytical skills to determine the answer to an issue?
- Able to verbally provide the reason/rationale for a patient care activity or intervention?
- Able to verbalize opportunities for improvement in patient care?
- Able to verbalize understanding of patient situations and intervene accordingly?
- Able to verbalize the difference between normal and abnormal findings?
- Able to question inconsistencies?

- Able to consider multiple ways to solve an issue?
- Able to demonstrate systematic patient assessment?
- Using all aspects of the nursing process (assessment, planning, intervention) and is able to verbalize comprehension of the different steps for their patient?
- Aware of and is utilizing applicable nursing standards for their patients?
- Aware of ethics codes and adheres to them?
- Able to prioritize and re-prioritize care?
- Able to make appropriate decisions?

## THE FIVE-MINUTE PRECEPTOR (5MP)

### Step 1: Get the Preceptee to Take a Stand

- State general, not specific, comments or questions about a patient care situation.
- Purposefully withhold information relevant to the case. *Example*: You could ask the preceptee in a given situation, "Tell me about what's happening with your patient." The preceptee will have to process the clinical information and communicate it to you. This information should include an interpretation of the clinical condition of the patient and the current patient situation.

### Step 2: Probe for Supporting Evidence

- After listening to the response the preceptee provided in step 1, begin to ask questions designed to "elicit evidence or rationale" (Bott, Mohide, & Lawlor, 2011) regarding the statement made by the preceptee. You are encouraging the preceptee to think about and express their knowledge of the situation.

**Fast Facts**

Probing questions will also assist the preceptor in assessing learning needs so that they can be addressed.

### Step 3: Teach General Rules

- As suggested by Bott et al. (2011), this step should include the sharing of a maximum of three points or "pearls" from you to the preceptee. Be sure that these are evidence based.

### Step 4: Reinforce the Positives

- Positive feedback is shared along with "rationale or explanations that reinforce the preceptee's strengths and competencies (knowledge, skills and/or attitudes), so that the positives can be applied reliably in future related situations" (Bott et al., 2011).

### Step 5: Correct Errors and Misinterpretations

- Provide constructive feedback (see Chapter 8, The Value of Feedback) intended to "help the preceptee improve understanding and future clinical performance" (Bott et al., 2011).

## CASE STUDY: USE OF THE FIVE-MINUTE PRECEPTOR

### Step 1: Get the Preceptee to Take a Stand

*Preceptor to preceptee*: "Tell me what's going on with your patient."

*Preceptee*: "I'm taking care of Ms. Smith. She had surgery for a small bowel obstruction yesterday and has a nasogastric tube in place to low wall suction. When I came in this morning, I noticed that there was no drainage from the NGT in the canister. It's almost 4 hours later and there is still no drainage present. The patient is complaining of nausea. I'm going to call the MD."

### Step 2: Probe for Supporting Evidence

*Preceptor*: "Tell me why you feel that you should call the MD at this time."

*Preceptee*: "Since Ms. Smith is only one day postop from GI surgery, there should be drainage from the NGT and there is not. This could indicate that the NGT is not functioning."

### Step 3: Teach General Rules

*Preceptor*: "For any patient with an NGT, you should assess the function of the tube and presence of suction material at the beginning of your shift and throughout. In the report, you should question the amount of drainage noted and the description from the shift before. You should check for bowel sounds and the presence of nausea and abdominal distention, which could indicate that there are stomach contents that are not being removed by suction. In NGTs like the

Salem Sump, you should hear a soft whistling sound from the blue pigtail, indicating that the tube is intact and working. You can insufflate air in order to push the tip of the tube away from the wall of the stomach; suction should start to work at that point. When you have done all of your assessments and found that the tube is not working, then you should call the MD."

### Step 4: Reinforce the Positives

*Preceptor*: "It is good that you noticed that no suction contents were present when you began your shift, and at this point you knew to focus on this aspect of the abdominal assessment."

### Step 5: Correct Errors or Misinterpretations

*Preceptor*: "First, before calling an MD, you should gather all the evidence you can to support your statement. This is true in any patient care situation. You may have called the MD too soon and not have done all you could to correct the situation and find a cause. Also, if you identify a patient care issue early, you should communicate your findings and begin to follow up immediately and not wait for several hours. Let me show you the unit policy on NGTs. There is also a computer-based educational summary on Salem Sump tubes I want to show you. Please review them and then we can talk about them."

## SBAR COMPETENCY

### Before Calling the MD, the Preceptee

- Assessed the patient
- Reviewed the chart for important information and read physician (MD) and RN notes
- Chose the appropriate MD to call
- Verified the patient's admitting diagnosis and prior history
- Verified the code status
- Verified allergies
- Noted intravenous (IV) fluids
- Noted significant lab work results
- Noted significant test results

Remind the preceptee that every SBAR report form is different depending on clinical area and facility. However, similar across all forms is the need for the RN to focus on the problem, to be concise in reporting, and to have all the information needed before calling the MD.

## S – Situation

- Nurse's name        Unit
- Patient's name       eoom #
- Inquires if the MD is familiar with this patient
- States the reason for their concern

## B – Background

- States the reason for the patient being in the hospital
- Lists current vital signs
- Lists the current pulse oximetry reading and the amount of $O_2$ the patient is receiving
- Notes the results of current physical assessment
- Notes if there is a change from past physical assessment
- Notes the presence of pain and the pain level
- Notes the patient's mental status and if this is a change from the previous report

## A – Assessment

- Verbalizes their assessment of the current situation
- Verbalizes what they feel may be happening with the patient or states that they are not sure what is occurring but the patient's status is deteriorating
- If necessary, explains that they feel the condition of the patient is severe or life-threatening

## R – Recommendation

- Notes what actions or orders from the MD they would like to see occur (medication, tests, lab work, EKG, CXR)
- Requests transfer to a critical care unit
- Notes if they require the MD to come to the unit
- Asks if the MD would like to be called back, and for what reason and in what time period
- Requests what assessments the MD would like repeated and in what time period (lab work, vital signs)

## EVIDENCE-BASED PRACTICE (EBP) GUIDELINES: HOW DO I KNOW IT IS EVIDENCE BASED?

### EBP Competencies

According to the Academy of Medical Surgical Nursing (AMSN), EBP should be one of the five competencies that all nurses should possess. Also according to the AMSN, all nurses should:

- Be able to verbalize where and how to find the best possible source of EBP for their specialty area
- Know how to formulate clear clinical questions
- Know how to search for relevant answers to the questions
- Determine when and how to integrate these new findings into practice

Find more information here: https://www.amsn.org/practice -resources/evidence-based-practice

### The Five As

In 2013, The University of North Carolina at Chapel Hill Health Sciences Library published the "Five As" that will help you to remember the EBN process:

1. **Ask**: Information needs from practice are converted into focused, structured questions.
2. **Acquire**: The focused questions are used as a basis for literature searching in order to identify relevant external evidence from research.
3. **Appraise**: The research evidence is critically appraised for validity.
4. **Apply**: The best available evidence is used alongside clinical expertise and the patient's perspective to plan care.
5. **Assess**: Performance is evaluated through a process of self-reflection, audit, or peer assessment.

For further information on these steps, please visit "The Five-Step Process" at www.lib.umn.edu/apps/instruction/ebp/ and the KT Clearinghouse at http://ktclearinghouse.ca/cebm/syllabi/nursing/ intro.

### RIME Tool in NP Education

#### Reporter—"What Is Happening?"

An NP student at the beginning of their education should be able to do the following. At the end of this stage, they should have mastered the requirements and be able to move on to the next stage.

- They are able to accurately review the patient record and collect data on their patient assignment.
- They should then be able to report (both verbally and in writing) their findings in a pre-clinical conference or when asked by the preceptor.
- They are expected to be able to explain the difference between what is important patient information and what is not important
- They are expected to know the difference between normal and abnormal patient findings.
- They should be able to recognize new patient problems.
- Their data collection and oral/written presentation should focus on the most important patient care issues to be prioritized.

#### Interpreter—"Why Is This Happening"

The next stage for the NP student is that of interpreter. At this stage they should be able to:

- Identify patient problems independently and to prioritize them
- Identify new patient problems as they occur
- Develop a differential diagnosis independently and justify what diagnosis they have chosen
- Interpret new and existing data

#### Manager—"What's Next?"

Only some NP students will meet this stage while still in school. However, all new NPs during their preceptorship should be able to:

- Develop and cite why they have chosen their diagnoses and their plan for each
- Decide what clinical action to take, such as what tests should be ordered. They are able to verbalize the rationale for their actions.
- Customize a plan of care based on the patient's current condition and preference

*Educator—"What Don't I Know"*

An NP with at least 2 years of experience should have mastered the three previous steps of reporting, interpreting, and managing. At the educator stage they should be able to

- Identify what they do not know
- Be self-directed
- Seek out the evidence-based reasoning for their actions
- Share their knowledge with other NPs or other members of the healthcare team
- Use their knowledge of nursing research to understand the limits and quality of evidence-based knowledge

## References

Alfaro-LeFebre, R. (2008). *Evidence-based approaches to promoting critical thinking.* Retrieved from www.alfaroteachsmart.com/powerpoint/h0-mln-austin-ctprogram08.pdf

Banning, M. (2006). Nursing research: Perspectives on crucial thinking. *British Journal of Nursing, 15*(8), 458–461. doi:10.12968/bjon.2006.15.8.20966

Bott, G., Mohide, E. A., & Lawlor, Y. (2011). A clinical teaching technique for nurse preceptors: The five minute preceptor. *Journal for Professional Nursing.* Retrieved from www.professionalnursing.org/article/S8755-7223(10)00119-5/pdf

Rubenfeld, M. G., & Scheffer, B. K. (2015). *Critical thinking tactics for nurses: Achieving the IOM competencies* (3rd ed.). Boston, MA: Jones & Bartlett Learning.

University of North Carolina at Chapel Hill Health Sciences Library. (2013). *Using evidence based practice.* Chapel Hill, NC: Author. Retrieved from http://guides.lib.unc.edu/ebn_practice

## Bibliography

Clair, E. RIME evaluation framework found on Pinterest. *Mayo Clinic Family Residency.*

Hendricson, W. D., & Kleffner, J. (2002). Assessing and helping challenging students: Part one, why do some students have difficulty learning? *Journal of Dental Education, 66*(1), 43–61.

# 17

# Concerns of the Preceptor and Case Studies

*As with any position, experience helps you gain insight. Each time you precept, you gain understanding and comfort with the routine; however, each time you precept, an issue may occur that you have never experienced before. Empathizing with the preceptee and remembering situations that you may have encountered yourself will help you understand and deal with new situations. As stated before, always remember that you are the advocate for the preceptee and, as such, you will guide them through new and difficult situations. Both of you will learn from them. Many of the scenarios discussed in this chapter are common to all clinical areas.*

After reading this chapter, the reader will be able to:

1. List steps to avoid a medication error
2. Describe how to care for a dying patient
3. Describe how to care for a patient who has expired
4. List common errors committed by a preceptee
5. Describe how to prevent errors

## SCENARIO 1: THE NURSE BEING USED AS STAFF BEFORE THE END OF ORIENTATION

You work on your shift as scheduled. The preceptee reports she has been given her own patient assignment and won't be working with you. The preceptee is upset but was told she did not have a choice. You are upset because you don't feel the preceptee is ready to function independently *and* you were not notified of the decision.

Using the new nurse as staff can occur at any time during orientation. If the preceptor is absent, the situation may be taken advantage of due to staffing issues, or nursing administration or staff may feel the preceptee has had "enough" orientation and is ready to be added to the schedule before the end of orientation. This often occurs without the permission or input of the preceptor or staff development educator and almost always without the preceptee's prior notification. This occurrence is inappropriate, and a hazard to the safety of the patients and the quality of care they receive.

The solution to this issue begins *before* start of the preceptor period.

- The orientation process itself must be respected by all involved, including administration, staff nurses, human resources, fellow educators, and the staffing office.
- All must "buy into" the fact that a positive orientation and the eventual long-term retention of the preceptee depend on a successful orientation process.
- The orientation schedule should be set and not deviated from. It should be arranged with the input of the unit manager, staff educator, preceptor, and preceptee.
- All must agree that the preceptee is not considered to be staff and that the staffing schedule should be formulated *without* the preceptee being considered as staff.
- All must agree that the preceptee is not a substitute for absent nurses or aides.
- The preceptee should work the same schedule as the preceptor.
- The preceptor should not have a patient assignment while orienting a new nurse

You are the advocate for the preceptee. It is your responsibility to speak for preceptees, since they may be afraid to speak for themselves.

## SCENARIO 2: MEDICATION ERROR

The preceptee comes to you after discovering they have committed a medication error.

According to Saintsing, Gibson, and Pennington (2011), 75% of new nurses commit a medication error, making it the most common error committed by the new nurse. Medication errors occur for a variety of reasons. The most common causes, according to the American Society of Health-System Pharmacists, include the following:

- Confusing strength designation on medication labels
- SALADs, or "sound-alike, look-alike drugs"
- Equipment failure or malfunction (e.g., intravenous [IV] pumps)
- Illegible handwriting
- Improper transcription
- Inaccurate dosage calculation
- Inadequately trained personnel
- Inappropriate abbreviations used in prescribing
- Labeling errors
- Excessive workloads of healthcare staff
- Lapses in performance (interruptions, phone calls, call lights)

Before preceptees administer medications, remind them they are the last line of defense in medication error prevention. Review with them how to prevent medication errors.

## How to Prevent a Medication Error

- Verify with the patient any allergies before administering a medication.
- Be familiar with all policies and procedures regarding medication administration in the facility. This includes medication order processing and administration times.
- Verify the identity of the patient following facility guidelines for the process.
- Verify all medication orders before the medication is administered.
- *Always* check the original order before administering the first dose of a medication.
- *Do not* administer the medication unless it is understood why the medication is being prescribed and that the order is correct.
- *Do not* borrow medications from another patient or other patient care unit. If an ordered medication was not sent by the pharmacy, do not circumvent and administer by borrowing it from elsewhere. There may be a reason the mediation was not sent (e.g., drug allergy or other contraindication). Call the pharmacy to investigate.
- Always question when large volumes (more than two of a tablet, capsule, vial, or amp) are to be administered.
- Always understand how to use medication administration devices (e.g., IV pumps) before using them. Never use them without understanding how they work.
- Always, always, always *stop* administering a medication when a patient questions what you are giving them. Ninety-nine times out of 100 the patient is correct that a medication is unfamiliar. Always check the original order.

## Medication Pass

- Presumably, the preceptee has passed a competency assessment for medication administration (e.g., by attending a Med Pass training program) and has administered medications prelicensure. It is still good practice for the preceptor to directly observe the nurse as they identify the patient and prepare and administer the medication in any form for the first time. This is done for several reasons:
  - First, although the preceptee may be an RN, they may not have had the opportunity to administer certain types of medication outside of a simulation environment.

- The second reason is for your acknowledgment the preceptee is knowledgeable about the process.
- If the preceptee is not competent during your observation, they should be referred back to the staff development/nursing education department.

- Ensure that the preceptee is following the rights of medication administration at all times and reinforce that by following these rights consistently, a medication error can be avoided.
- It may helpful to review and follow the medication administration checklist (also a good review for the preceptor!) in Chapter 16, Preceptorship Competency Forms and Clinical Tools.
- Review the process of reporting the medication error with the preceptee. Have the preceptee complete all required documentation and activities as per unit or facility protocol.
- Understand and empathize with the fact that the preceptee will be very anxious and fearful.
- Emphasize to the preceptee that medication errors should be reported according to the method prescribed by the facility without fear of reprisal.
- Allow the preceptee to call the patient's MD and any other personnel as outlined in facility policy.

**Fast Facts**

Medication errors can be the fault of the *system* and not just due to the actions of an individual. Be proactive in reporting systemic issues you feel may lead (or have already led) to errors.

## SCENARIO 3: THE DYING PATIENT

One of the patients in your assignment is dying. The preceptee appears anxious and nervous and verbalizes that they feel unprepared to care for the patient.

Be empathic and remember what it was like the first time you cared for a dying patient. You probably felt nothing would help you prepare to emotionally support the dying patient. Many nurses have an image of what they should do in response to the death of their patient but feel unable to meet those expectations during the care of the patient. Allow the preceptee to speak about their feelings and experience their own grief. Encourage the preceptee to deal with the death within their own belief system.

The preceptee should:

- Honor the psychological needs of the patient.
- Let patients decide who they wish to have at their side.
- Remain at the bedside of the dying patient if there are no significant others present. Unfortunately, many times in the "real world" of nursing today, this is not possible. It should be. Consider the person who must die alone and if this occurs on your unit, work to change it.
- Utilize the therapeutic technique of listening. Allow the patient to verbalize their fears, anxieties, and wishes.
- Know that the nurse's presence with the patient is also therapeutic.
- Use touch to convey feelings of care and concern.
- Honor the spiritual needs of the patient.
- Allow the patient's family to place religious articles near the patient. Administer medications recommended or ordered by hospice to decrease anxiety and ease breathing. If the preceptee is reluctant to do so because they feel these medications will hasten the patient's death, provide reassurance that the mediations will decrease anxiety and provide for a comfortable death. It may be helpful for the preceptee to speak to a hospice representative or attend hospice education.

**Fast Facts**

Explain the nurse is also caring for the family of the dying patient and should advocate for the family as well.

Familiarize the preceptee with the signs of imminent death and what they indicate. Review the details of care to be provided for a dying patient and any unit policies and procedures.

Care of the dying patient consists of the following:

- Allowing the patient to maintain as much independence as possible
- Providing dim lighting in the patient's room (A darkened room may frighten the patient.)
- Providing eye care to eliminate the accumulation of secretions

- Talking to the patient and verbalizing what actions they are taking in the care of the patient (The patient may not respond, but they may hear, and speaking to the patient will help to allay fears by offering reassurance and comfort.)
- Providing oral care to prevent the mouth and lips from becoming dry and cracked
- Keeping the mouth and lips moist by rinsing with water, using saliva substitute, or applying an oral moisturizing gel or lip moisturizer
- Providing a cool-mist humidifier in the room
- Avoiding mouthwashes containing alcohol and lemon glycerin swabs, which cause dryness
- Providing care to the membranes of the nose, which can become dry from supplemental oxygen
- Providing skin care, including frequent bathing and interventions to prevent skin breakdown
- Changing the patient's position frequently, avoiding skin-to-skin contact, and using pillows to maintain body position

## SCENARIO 4: THE PATIENT WHO HAS EXPIRED

A patient within your assignment has expired. The preceptee has not experienced a death before and is unsure of the care to provide.

Many nurses are uncomfortable caring for the body after death; this is natural. When the preceptee encounters this situation:

- Encourage the preceptee to perform postmortem care, but do not leave them alone with the patient.
- If facility RNs may pronounce the patient dead, have the preceptee with you to follow and perform this procedure.
- Allow the preceptee to verbalize their feelings, and explain that this is the last act of care the nurse provides for the patient and family.
- Ascertain whether the family is coming to the facility for a last goodbye, if they were not at the bedside when the patient expired.
- Maintain standard health care precautions.
- Assist the preceptee in cleaning the patient's body while promoting dignity.
- Explain to the preceptee that to deal with stress, many nurses talk to the patient while they complete their care.
- Place the patient in a natural position.
- Maintain low lighting in the room.

- Ensure that the patient's room is cleaned and used medical items are disposed of or removed.
- Gather, pack, and store all personal belongings according to facility policy.
- Place the patient's dentures in the mouth, if able.

## SCENARIO 5: THEY "JUST DON'T GET IT"

The preceptee fails to correctly perform a new skill despite reviewing the provided literature and observing the preceptor.

Understand that adults learn in different ways. Some must read about the skill, some must have the skill demonstrated, and so on.

- Review with the staff development educator what equipment is available in your facility to address clinical skills.
- Also communicate with staff development or school faculty about the preceptee's difficulty.
- If the preceptee is a student, follow necessary protocol, including communication and documentation, and refer the preceptee back to the nursing skills lab at their school. The skills lab should then provide documentation that the student has mastered the skill before they return to the clinical area.
- To consider all areas of adult learning in a new nurse in cooperation with staff development protocols, have the preceptee read about the skill, view a prescribed video on the procedure, observe while the skill is performed in a simulated environment, and then perform the skill again in a simulated environment. Allow the preceptee to repeat the skill in a simulated environment as often as necessary (as long they are making progress each time). Measure the preceptee's performance utilizing a competency assessment for documentation purposes.
- Nonmastery of a skill should be referred to the staff development educator.

## SCENARIO 6: A PATIENT CARE ERROR

Your preceptee has been providing care to the same assignment over several days. Both you and they are feeling confident in their progression, enough that you allow them to work with minimal supervision.

At one point during the shift, they come to you and explain an error in care has occurred.

According to Saintsing et al. (2011), between 49% and 53% of new nurses are involved in errors of nursing care. The majority of errors are medication errors (see Scenario 2), improper patient supervision (most often leading to patient falls), and delay in patient care (this includes failure to administer medications as prescribed, as well as failure to recognize and failure to intervene in relation to patient care). Other errors noted by Saintsing and colleagues include:

- Improper documentation
- Inadequate communication with MDs
- Not following facility policy and procedures
- Increased wound infection rate
- Not understanding how equipment works
- Increased mortality

Causes of preceptee errors according to Saintsing and colleagues include:

- Not asking for help when it is needed
- Time limitations (inability to complete a task)
- Poor critical thinking skills
- Poor time management
- Poor prioritization
- Inability to convert school learning to "real world" scenarios

Although not foolproof, the following strategies may assist the preceptee in avoiding errors:

- Anticipate that there will be errors and problems and attempt to be one step ahead of the process.
- Gradually increase the number of patients in the preceptee's assignment from the number they took care of during school clinical to a full assignment. Do not advance the number of patients until confidence with the original number is attained.
- Encourage the preceptee to ask questions *at any time*, and be open to questions regarding all aspects of patient care including equipment use and procedures.
- Encourage critical thinking (see Chapter 4, The Challenging Student).

"A good scare is worth more to a man than good advice."
—E. W. Howe.

## SCENARIO 7: A "CONTROLLED SCARE"

Howe's quote has great relevance for nursing. Sometimes showing
the preceptee how to complete a skill or care for a patient will have
an impact, and sometimes it won't. What may have a greater impact
than demonstrating care is the "controlled scare." Just as a full medication error will never be forgotten (or repeated) by the seasoned
nurse, the controlled scare that raises an at-risk situation will not be
forgotten. Below are characteristics of the controlled scare:

- Allow the preceptee to complete a skill or action under close
  supervision.
- If you observe that an error will occur (one that will not place the
  patient in danger), allow the preceptee to complete the skill to the
  point of causing potential harm and immediately stop the preceptee.
- Be prepared to complete the procedure yourself.
- Speak to the preceptee in a private area (never in front of the
  patient or staff), review what you have observed, and question
  the preceptee utilizing the critical thinking questions found in
  Chapter 4, The Challenging Student.

**Example of a controlled scare:** Observe the preceptee pouring medications for one patient that are meant for another. Allow the procedure to continue, to the point when the preceptee attempts to identify
the patient and discovers (hopefully) it is the wrong patient. Stop the
preceptee, excuse the preceptee and yourself from the patient's room,
and go to a private area to discuss, utilizing critical thinking, what just
occurred. Have the preceptee begin again and complete the procedure.

## SCENARIO 8: PRECEPTOR BURNOUT

You have been asked to precept yet *another* new RN for your unit.
Although you love to teach, you are tired and just want to care for

your patients. It's beginning to seem as if there is a revolving door at the end of the unit, as new staff just come and go.

Preceptor burnout is a very real phenomenon. It is caused by a variety of factors including:

- Lack of training in how to be a preceptor
- Lack of monetary compensation for precepting
- Lack of advance notice of a precepting assignment
- The feeling that the preceptor will not be able to properly precept another nurse while still caring for their own assignment of patients
- Added workload and additional responsibility

Strategies for how to prevent burnout rest with the facility where the preceptor works. Facility administration (including non-nursing administration), should acknowledge the importance of a professionally organized and presented preceptorship program in the education and retention of nursing staff. If the preceptor is involved with the evaluation of the program, the following should be suggested:

- Reward preceptors either monetarily or with other forms of recognition.
- Either develop or allow nurses to attend preceptor workshops.
- Include precepting on clinical ladder steps.
- Encourage support from clinical managers and administration.
- Share the importance of the preceptor role with other members of the staff.
- Encourage staff development support, including simulation and education on cultural differences and learning styles. Clinical educators are also needed to support the preceptor and answer any immediate questions or address any issues.
- Allow the preceptor to meet the nurse they will be precepting, providing advance notice and including them on the decision process during preceptorship.

## References

Saintsing, D., Gibson, L. M., & Pennington, A. (2011). The novice nurse and clinical decision making: How to avoid errors. *Journal of Nursing Management, 19*, 354–359. Retrieved from www.academia.edu/1522220/The_novice_nurse_and_clinical_decision-making_how_to_avoid_errors

# Index

advanced practice nurse (APRN)
preceptee, 118–124
role, 120
preceptor for, 120–122
barriers during preceptorship,
122–124
ANA (American Nurses
Association) Decision Tree
for Delegation, 110
assessment and planning, 110
communication, 111
right supervision, 111–112
observation and feedback, 112
ANA (American Nurses
Association) Scope and
Standards of Practice, 21
autonomy, 19

Bachelor's Degree, importance of,
181–183
BEER method. *See* Behavior, Effect,
Expectations, and Results
Behavior, Effect, Expectations,
and Results (BEER) method,
102
bully, how to deal with, 160–162
bullying in nursing, 159–162
causes, 159
effects, 159–160
targets of, 160

care, missing, 82–83
case studies 202–211
Scenario 1 – The nurse being
used as staff before end of
orientation, 202
Scenario 2 – Medication error,
203
Scenario 3 – The dying patient,
205–207
Scenario 4 – The patient who has
expired, 207–208
Scenario 5 – They "just don't get
it", 208
Scenario 6 – A patient care error,
208–209
Scenario 7 – The "controlled
scare", 210
Scenario 8 – Preceptor burnout,
210–211
certification, 180
clinical day, 63
before the first clinical day, 63–65
how the preceptor can minimize
stress/anxiety, 65–68
clinical teaching strategies for the
novice learner, 33–34
competence, 34–36
conscious, 35
stages of, 34–36
unconscious, 35

consciously competent, 46–47
  pre and post care, 55
  use of positive comments during,
    55–56
conflict 153–156
  causes, 156–157
  dealing with, 154, 155–156
  defined 153–154
  good vs. bad, 154
cognitive staffing, 83–85
critical thinking, 56
  characteristics, 51
  defined, 50–51
  habits, 51
  how not to promote, 58–59
  nursing process, 52–54
  questioning, 52
  teaching style to promote, 52,
    57–58
  thinking ahead, 56
  thinking in action, 56
  thinking back, 56–57
  traditional thinking, 59
Critical Thinking Evaluation
    Checklist, 193–194
curriculum vitae (CV), 174
conferences with preceptee, 55–56

debriefing, 87
delegation, 106–110
  five rights of, 108–110
  incorrect, 107
  preceptor/preceptee, 107
document review, 54–55

ethics and moral reasoning, 144–145
  "teaching" ethics, 145
evidence based practice, 60
  and competence, 198
  in delegation, 113
  "The 5 A's", 198
expert and novice, difference
    between, 41

feedback 98
  constructive/performance
    improvement, 98–100

sandwich, 101
  when provided, 98–99
"Fail to Fail", 140–142
feedback, 92
  delivery do's and don'ts, 93–96
  effective delivery, 97–98
  follow up, 97
  functions of, 92
  negative, 92
  poor nurse educators and, 92
  positive, 93, 100–101
  strong nurse educators and, 92
"Five Minute Preceptor", The, 58,
    194–195
  case student, 195–196
"Forces of Magnetism", 18

"I don't know!", 32
incompetence, 34
  conscious, 34
  unconscious, 34
information, preceptor unable to
    retrieve, 91
Initial Organization Review
    Checklist, 191–193
interdisciplinary relationships, 20

knowledge, poorly integrated,
    41–43

learner types 30–31
  auditory, 30
  kinesthetic, 30–31
  visual, 30
learner, novice, 32
learning, adult 29–30
  principles, 29–30
  types, 30
learning difficulties, 6 factors
    related to 40–41
  academic environment, 40
  affective component, 40
  cognition, 40
  distraction, 40
  medical condition, underlying,
    40
  study habits, 40

learning disability, undiagnosed, 43
  signs of, 43
learning, generational differences
  in, 36–37
  baby boomer, 36
  Generation X, 36
  Generation Y, 37
  Generation Z, 37
  veterans, 36
learning, stages of, 34
learning, three domains of, 31
  affective, 31
  cognitive, 31
  psychomotor, 31

management style, 19
medication administration, 189–191
mentor, 7
  characteristics of successful
    (great) mentor, 10–11
  key responsibilities of, 9
  nursing student, 8–9
  positive impact of, 9–10
Myers Briggs personality
  assessment, 26

nurse residency programs, 183–184
nurses as teachers, 20
nursing, image of, 20
nursing leadership, quality of, 18

One Minute Preceptor, The,
  124–125
  get a commitment, 124
  give guidance about errors or
    omissions, 125
  probe for supporting evidence,
    124
  reinforce what was well done, 124
  teach a general principle, 124

performing unsuccessfully, 135
personnel policies and programs, 19
PET. See Prime, Partition, Praise,
  Empathy, Expectations,
  Teach, Help and Model
phone skills, 79–81

portfolio, 174
  development, 174
  electronic, 179–180
  growth and development, 175
  professional, 175
  showcasing, 178–179
  steps, 176
post conference, 87
preceptee
  accelerated BSN, 116
  begin at the beginning, 128
  challenges, 117
  distracted, 45–46
  failure to seek assistance, 143
  failure to recognize patient
    distress, 143
  how to assist, 117–118
  knowledge deficit, 143
  novice, as, 32
  struggling, 128
  unethical, 142
  unprofessional, 142
  unsafe, 142
  what they require from educators
    and preceptors, 117
  who requires additional education
    or remediation, 143
preceptor, online courses, 26
preceptor
  advocate, 7
  ANCC (American Nurses
    Credentialing Center)
    Magnet Status standards, 18
  behavior associated with, 6
  burnout, causes of, 24
  candidate focus, 18
  competency, 21
  curriculum, 23–24
  education needed, 20
  encounters with preceptee, 28
  evaluation of, 24
  Ineffectual, behavior associated
    with, 4–5
  Knowledge needed, 20
  leader, manager, 6
  policies concerning, 23
  primary roles of, 21

preceptor (*continued*)
  retention, 24–25
  role model, 7
  selection instrument, 21
  selection of, 17–18
  skills needed, 20
preceptor – preceptee conflict,
    158–159
preceptorship
  conditions, 9
  establishment phase, 11–12
  less than ideal conditions, 16
  phases of, 11
  quality clinical in, 45
  rewards, 16–17
  working phase, 12–13
Prime, Partition, Praise, Empathy,
    Expectations, Teach, Help
    and Model (PET), 46–47
prioritization, 86–88
  CURE, 88–89
problem personality, 103
professional development, 20
professional models of care, 19
psychological reaction, 155
  fight (aggressor), 155
  flight (passive), 155
  unintentional, 155

quality of care, 19
quality improvement, 19

rapid response team, 50
reality shock, 164
  causes of 164–165
  honeymoon phase, 165
  how to help, 169–171
  recovery, 167–168
  resolution, 168–160
  shock, 166–167
Reporter, Interpreter, Manager,
    Educator (RIME), 125

in NP education, 199–200
  the reason for, 125
resume, 174
RIME. *See* Reporter, Interpreter,
    Manager, Educator
routinization, 86
  when to use, 86

SBAR. *See* Situation, Background,
    Assessment, Recommendation
Scope and Standards of Practice,
    American Nurses
    Association, 21
setting the preceptee up to fail, 146
  how to avoid, 136
shift organization, 68–71
study habits, bad, 44–45
Situation, Background, Assessment,
    Recommendation (SBAR)
  and competency, 196–197
  description of, 78–79
SUCCESS, 128–134
  See it early, 128–129
  Clarify the situation with the
    preceptee, 130–131
  Contract with the preceptee for
    success, 131–133
  Evaluate the preceptee regularly,
    133
  Summarize the performance, 134
  Understand the preceptees point
    of view and feelings, 130
successful preceptorship, 134

"things", how they get missed, 81

unsafe practice
  how to prevent, 145–148
  what to do, 146–147
unsuccessful preceptorship,
    134–135

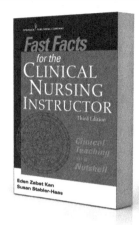
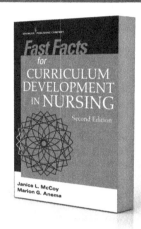
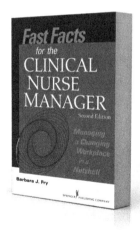
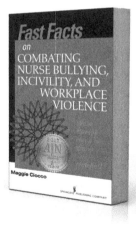

Printed in the United States
by Baker & Taylor Publisher Services